Immunology and Immune System Disorders

Medicine & Health
New York

Immunology and Immune System Disorders

The Dangers of Allergic Asthma
Jesús Miguel García-Menaya, PhD, MD (Editor)
2023. ISBN: 979-8-88697-553-6 (Hardcover)
2023. ISBN: 979-8-88697-724-0 (eBook)

Signaling Pathways of the Immune System
Kenan Demir, PhD (Editor)
Mustafa Usanmaz, MD (Editor)
2023. ISBN: 979-8-88697-603-8 (Softcover)
2023. ISBN: 979-8-88697-681-6 (eBook)

Mast Cells and their Role in Health and Disease
Ana I. Faustino, PhD (Editor), Paula A. Oliveira, PhD (Editor)
2022. ISBN: 978-1-68507-628-3 (Softcover)
2022. ISBN: 978-1-68507-690-0 (eBook)

Cytokines and Diseases
Kenan Demir, MD (Editor)
Selim Görgün, MD (Editor)
Bahar Uslu, MD, PhD (Editor)
2022. ISBN: 979-8-88697-214-6 (Hardcover)
2022. ISBN: 979-8-88697-322-8 (eBook)

The Innate Immune System in Health and Disease: From the Lab Bench Work to Its Clinical Implications. Volume 1
Jorge Morales-Montor, PhD (Editor)
2022. ISBN: 978-1-68507-507-1 (Hardcover)
2022. ISBN: 978-1-68507-644-3 (eBook)

More information about this series can be found at
https://novapublishers.com/product-category/series/immunology-and-immune-system-disorders/

Chenguang Shen
Yang Yang
and Minghui Yang
Editors

Neutralizing Antibodies and their Role in Health and Disease

nova
Medicine & Health
New York

https://doi.org/10.52305/CJKN3850

NOTICE TO THE READER

Library of Congress Cataloging-in-Publication Data

ISBN: 979-8-89113-541-3 (Hardcover)
ISBN: 979-8-89113-701-1 (eBook)

Published by Nova Science Publishers, Inc. † New York

Contents

Preface

As of July 2023, 209 monoclonal antibody drugs have been approved by the FDA for marketing use, which are widely distributed in the fight against immune diseases, infectious diseases, and neurological and metabolic diseases. In this book, we introduce current monoclonal drug development techniques, delivery and therapeutic application of neutralizing antibodies, development and application of anti-inflammatory factor monoclonal antibodies, research progress and prospect of monoclonal antibodies against human infectious diseases (including SARS-CoV-2, Enterovirus, Herpesvirus, Hepatitis Virus, and Orthopoxvirus), and the research and applications of nanobodies in human infectious diseases. Most of the content of this book is aimed at viral infectious diseases that are widespread and seriously endanger human health. For example, SARS-CoV-2 continues to circulate the world. Enteroviral infections continue to cause morbidity and mortality in susceptible individuals worldwide. Hepatitis viruses continue to constitute a significant global health threat that results in substantial morbidity and mortality; Herpesviruses lead to significant health challenges, notably through conditions like herpes, varicella, zoster, mononucleosis, and various cancers including Kaposi's sarcoma, nasopharyngeal carcinoma, and lymphoma. This book provides valuable insights for designing next-generation monoclonal antibodies.

Chapter 1- Monoclonal antibodies (MAbs) are homogeneous antibodies produced by a single B-cell against only one antigenic epitope, and their main biological functions include neutralization of antigens, modulation of cellular phagocytosis, activation of complement, and mediation of cytotoxicity. Because of their specificity, long serum half-life, high affinity and immune effector function have transformed them from scientific tools to novel targeted drugs for treating important human diseases. As of July 2023, 209 monoclonal antibody drugs have been approved by the FDA for marketing use, which are widely distributed in oncology, immune diseases, infectious diseases, and neurological and metabolic diseases. After more than 30 years of research and development, monoclonal antibodies have gone through the process of mouse-derived monoclonal antibodies, chimeric antibodies, humanized antibodies, and fully human monoclonal antibodies. Their antibody discovery platforms have achieved a variety of biotechnological breakthroughs, such as the more widely used hybridoma technology, phage display technology, single B-cell gene amplification technology and B-cell stimulation and culture technology, as well as genetically modified mouse technology, ribosome demonstration technology, ribosome demonstration technology and yeast cell demonstration technology are also used for the discovery and preparation of MAbs.

Chapter 2 - Neutralizing antibodies (NAbs) have been extensively employed as promising prophylactic and therapeutic reagents for preventing or treating infections, cancers, and inflammation-related diseases. However, their effectiveness is generally limited by short half-life, poor biodistribution, low bioavailability, and potential immunogenicity. To address these challenges, developing delivery systems to enhance biocompatibility, reduce swift immune clearance in vivo, and enable effective and targeted delivery of NAbs is critical. Herein, the authors provide an overview of the state-of-the-art achievements in the delivery strategies and therapeutic application of NAbs. First, a brief description of the mechanism of action and classification of NAbs is provided. Next, the authors highlight the examination of literature pertinent to the delivery platforms, routes of administration, and therapeutic applications of NAbs. The authors hope this review can provide valuable insights for designing next-generation NAbs that integrate precise delivery strategies and administration routes tailored to specific therapeutic needs.

Chapter 3 - Enteroviral infections continue to cause morbidity and mortality in susceptible individuals worldwide. However, effective antiviral drugs or vaccines remain lacking in targeting most circulating enteroviruses. Antibody-mediated immunity plays a crucial role in preventing and limiting enteroviral infections. This review primarily focuses on enteroviruses that have caused recent endemics, including poliovirus, enterovirus A71 (EV-A71), coxsackievirus and rhinovirus. Additionally, the authors provide an insightful analysis of the structural mechanisms underlying virus neutralization. The mechanisms underlying the neutralization of enteroviruses by type-specific antibodies have been demonstrated to target different steps of the viral infection cascade, including blocking virion-receptor interactions, inducing premature uncoating of virions via functional mimicry, or destabilizing the capsid and inducing virion disruption. These type-specific neutralizing antibodies have demonstrated the ability to target multiple antigenic loops, recognize distinct viral conformations, and offer protective effects solely against a limited subset of viruses. Moreover, this review also discusses recent advances in the relative importance of Fc-dependent effector functions and the structural rearrangements that occur during the antibody cocktail. These findings offer valuable insights into the potential mechanisms underlying enterovirus neutralization.

Chapter 4 - Herpesviruses lead to significant health challenges, notably through conditions like herpes, varicella, zoster, mononucleosis, and various cancers including Kaposi's sarcoma, nasopharyngeal carcinoma, and lymphoma. Yet, no approved treatments explicitly target the initial infections of herpesviruses. The herpesviruses' cell entry mechanism relies on the coordinated action of several glycoproteins and involves multiple host cell receptors. Glycoprotein B (gB) is essential for membrane fusion and gets activated by the entry complex, primarily formed of gH and gL. Given the central role of this entry complex and the fusogen in herpesvirus infections, antibodies neutralizing targeting the key epitopes on these glycoproteins offer a promising strategy to counteract herpesvirus infections.

Chapter 5 - Hepatitis viruses constitute a significant global health threat, resulting in substantial morbidity and mortality on a global scale. The pursuit of effective therapeutic strategies to combat hepatitis virus infections remains a paramount objective within the realm of medical research. Among the promising candidates, neutralizing antibodies (NAbs) have emerged as noteworthy therapeutic agents due to their capacity to impede viral entry and replication. This chapter provides an overview of recent advancements in the investigation of NAbs targeting various hepatitis viruses, encompassing hepatitis A, B, C, D, and E viruses. The authors' discourse delves into elucidating the mechanisms underlying neutralization, as well as their practical applications in the therapeutic domain. Additionally, the authors shed light on the challenges inherent in this research area and delineate the prospective trajectories for future exploration.

Chapter 6 - The re-emergence and spread of monkeypox (Mpox) worldwide poses a severe threat to the health and safety of the global population. This outlines the epidemiological characteristics of monkeypox, the pathological features of monkeypox virus, and the immune response following monkeypox infection, which may help raise awareness of monkeypox virus. In addition, it focuses on summarizing the key proteins of variola virus and the current development of neutralizing antibodies, providing a reference for the subsequent development of specific treatments and vaccines for monkeypox.

Chapter 7 - Variants of severe acute respiratory syndrome coronavirus 2 (SARS-CoV-2) continue to emerge and spread worldwide. Billions of vaccines against SARS-CoV-2 have been administered globally, effectively reducing the morbidity and mortality of coronavirus disease 2019 (COVID-19). The COVID-19 pandemic is wreaking havoc on public health and the global economy. One of the strategies to combat COVID-19 is the development of vaccines with broad-spectrum-neutralizing antibodies for prophylaxis and treatment. Anti-SARS-CoV-2 neutralizing antibodies are important to prevent infections and clear the virus, which is the key to offering long-term immunity. In addition, antiviral antibodies do not always have protective effects. The emergence of SARS-CoV-2 immune escape variants has contributed to the greater importance of vaccine design strategies and antibody-mediated therapies. A few antibodies are currently in preclinical and clinical development, and a few have been approved for emergency therapy. In this chapter, the current development status of anti-SARS-CoV-2 neutralizing antibodies was reviewed, and the focus was placed on their targets, mechanisms, and taxonomic characteristics. Additionally, severe challenges and possible future directions for neutralizing antibodies were discussed to guide the rational design of next-generation vaccines.

Chapter 8 - This chapter discusses the systemic inflammatory pathway in severe COVID-19 patients and explores whether the inflammatory factor antibodies could be a therapeutic option for severe COVID-19 patients. As IL-6 and IFN-γ are the critical factors in systemic inflammatory reactions, the relevant antibodies are potential choices.

Chapter 9 - Infectious diseases, triggered by pathogenic microorganisms, have the potential to lead to global crises. Beyond enduring infectious illnesses such as malaria and dengue fever, recent malevolent outbreaks of diseases like Neocon, Ebola, SARS-CoV, MERS-CoV, and SARS-CoV-2 have accelerated the search for more effective and accessible methods for improved diagnosis and treatment. Among the various avenues explored, antibodies have gained significant attention owing to their favorable structural characteristics and versatile applications. Nanobodies, also referred to as single domain-based VHHs and derived from heavy-chain only IgG antibodies found in the Camillidae family, can stably bind to antigens and offer a host of advantages such as high stability, pronounced hydrophilicity, and ease of expression and modification. These attributes allow them to directly target antigen epitopes or be engineered into multivalent nanobodies or nanobody fusion proteins to wield therapeutic effects. This paper provides an in-depth examination of the methods used to construct nanobodies and explores their potential functions, summarizing the current progress of research in the field and underscoring their diverse applications in the management and understanding of human infectious diseases.

Chapter 1

Monoclonal Antibody Development Technology for Important Human Diseases

Linlin Zhai*
and Chenguang Shen†
BSL-3 Laboratory (Guangdong), Guangdong Provincial Key Laboratory of Tropical Disease Research, School of Public Health, Southern Medical University, Guangzhou, People's Republic of China

Abstract

Monoclonal antibodies (MAbs) are homogeneous antibodies produced by a single B-cell against only one antigenic epitope, and their main biological functions include neutralization of antigens, modulation of cellular phagocytosis, activation of complement, and mediation of cytotoxicity. Because of their specificity, long serum half-life, high affinity and immune effector function have transformed them from scientific tools to novel targeted drugs for treating important human diseases. As of July 2023, 209 monoclonal antibody drugs have been approved by the FDA for marketing use, which are widely distributed in oncology, immune diseases, infectious diseases, and neurological and metabolic diseases. After more than 30 years of research and development, monoclonal antibodies have gone through the process of mouse-derived monoclonal antibodies, chimeric antibodies, humanized antibodies, and fully human monoclonal antibodies. Their antibody discovery platforms have achieved a variety of biotechnological breakthroughs, such as the more widely used hybridoma technology, phage display technology, single B-cell gene amplification technology

---

* Corresponding Author's Email: zll15649856209@163.com.
† Corresponding Author's Email: a124965468@smu.edu.cn.

In: Neutralizing Antibodies and their Role in Health and Disease
Editors: Chenguang Shen, Yang Yang and Minghui Yang
ISBN: 979-8-89113-541-3

and B-cell stimulation and culture technology, as well as genetically modified mouse technology, ribosome demonstration technology, ribosome demonstration technology and yeast cell demonstration technology are also used for the discovery and preparation of MAbs.

Keywords: monoclonal antibody discovery technology, b-cell culture technology, *in vivo* and *in vitro* evaluation of neutralizing antibodies, antibody humanization

Introduction

Monoclonal antibodies are one of the most important biological tools in molecular biology, biochemistry and medicine [1]. Due to their high specificity and sensitivity, monoclonal antibodies have been successfully used in diagnostic, therapeutic and targeted drug delivery systems for infectious diseases, cancers, autoimmune diseases and metabolic and hormonal disorders. The mechanism of action of antibody drugs mainly includes direct antibody action, ADCC/CDC, immunomodulation by targeting immune checkpoints, inhibition of receptor-ligand binding and modulatory effects [2]. Among them, monoclonal antibodies are the most direct and effective way to treat pathogenic infections, especially in virulent infectious diseases, and therapeutic fully human monoclonal antibodies targeting Ebola and HIV viruses are currently available [3, 4]. Thus, monoclonal antibodies have a wide range of applications in the biomedical field.

Antibiotic drugs are classified based on their host sources, including mouse-derived, rabbit-derived, humanized, and fully human antibodies. Early monoclonal antibodies were all mouse-derived and produced through hybridoma technology [5]. Hybridoma technology is convenient, simple, and low-cost. Still, mouse-derived antibodies can be recognized by the human immune system, causing human solid anti-mouse antibody responses, which generally require humanization through genetic engineering methods. Rabbit-derived antibodies have advantages over mouse-derived antibodies, such as high affinity and sensitivity. However, as ABcam holds the patent for the rabbit myeloma partner cell line 240W, rabbit-derived antibodies are generally obtained using phage display or single B cell gene amplification technologies [6]. Compared to antibodies from other species, fully human monoclonal antibodies have the advantage of having gene sequences entirely derived from humans, resulting in low immunogenicity and minimal side effects. Therefore, fully human monoclonal antibodies have become the main direction for the future development of monoclonal antibodies [7]. The leading technologies for rapidly preparing fully human monoclonal antibodies include phage display, single B cell PCR technology, and memory cell in vitro culture technology. Among them, memory B cell in vitro culture technology retains naturally paired variable regions of heavy and light chains, enabling rapid screening of neutralizing or specific human antibodies for research and development purposes. It has the advantages of short development cycles, high genetic diversity, low cost, and high success rates, making it an ideal method for screening human antibodies [8].

This chapter will review widely used methods for producing and humanizing monoclonal antibodies and describe their preparation processes and advantages and disadvantages. The focus of this chapter is on B cell in vitro culture technology. Using neutralizing antibodies as an example, this chapter will describe the method's processes for rapid screening of neutralizing antibodies, in vitro and in vivo evaluation of neutralizing antibodies, antigen epitope mapping, and virus neutralization mechanism identification.

Analytical Framework

Hybridoma Technology

Milstein and Kohler first described the production of monoclonal antibodies in mice through hybridoma technology. This method is based on the fusion of B cells isolated from an immunized animal with a myeloma partner cell, followed by screening and identifying specific hybridoma cell lines that can continuously secrete specific antibodies while proliferating indefinitely *in vitro*. As hybridoma technology is the basis for monoclonal antibody development, this section provides an overview of this technology.

The primary process for hybridoma technology includes animal immunization, cell fusion, hybridoma cell selection and cultivation, etc. (Figure 1) [9]. Animal immunization considers the immunogen and immunization strategy. Purified recombinant proteins are usually used as immunogens and can generate antibodies against different antigen epitopes. Different laboratories adopt different immunization strategies, typically relying on repeated stimulation of the antigen to enhance specific immune responses and to promote their maturation [10]. Cell fusion is the basis of hybridoma technology, which can be achieved using various techniques such as chemical fusion (with polyethylene glycol), viral (Sendai virus) or electric fusion. After fusion, cells are resuspended in selective culture media containing hypoxanthine, aminopterin, and thymidine (HAT), which blocks de novo DNA synthesis and allows cell survival only through a salvage pathway where hypoxanthine and thymidine are incorporated into DNA via hypoxanthine-guanine phosphoribosyltransferase (HGPRT). The parental myeloma cells will die in a selective medium due to HGPRT deficiency, while the unfused B cells cannot proliferate *in vitro* and fail to survive. Only the hybridoma cells formed by cell fusion can grow in the HAT medium. The cells from the fusion step are then distributed into 96-well plates containing HAT medium for cultivation for 10-14 days until cell clusters form in the wells. Positive clones can be identified by specific antibody screening using an enzyme-linked immunosorbent assay (ELISA), and then single monoclonal hybridoma cells that can continuously secrete antibodies can be immediately subcloned, amplified, and cryopreserved in this group. Positive clones typically contain more than one stable hybridoma cell line, so additional subcloning is required to obtain a single hybridoma cell line that secretes only one antibody. This is usually achieved through simple and easy-to-use limited dilution techniques [11]. After the hybridoma cells that produce specific antibodies are isolated, cloned, and stored in a library, the cells can be amplified or ascites can be prepared to produce antibodies.

With the advancement of technology, a new hybridoma screening technology, the Cellcelector automated cell screening system, has been widely used. This method uses semi-solid culture to grow cells into individual and independent, dispersed, and immobile single clones. Fluorescent halo-like substances are formed in the clone cells after adding a fluorescent-labeled clone detection reagent and capturing the target antibody. The production ratio of antibodies can be calculated as a quality coefficient by comparing the size of the halo diameter in the clone cells and the surrounding cells. The mechanical arm and picker can automatically pick the cell clone with the highest quality coefficient to obtain the highest antibody-producing clone. As the latest generation technology, the Cellcelector automated cell screening system has advantages such as high throughput, automation, efficiency, programmability, quantification, archiving and traceability, which can shorten the development cycle and reduce costs (Figure 2) [12, 13].

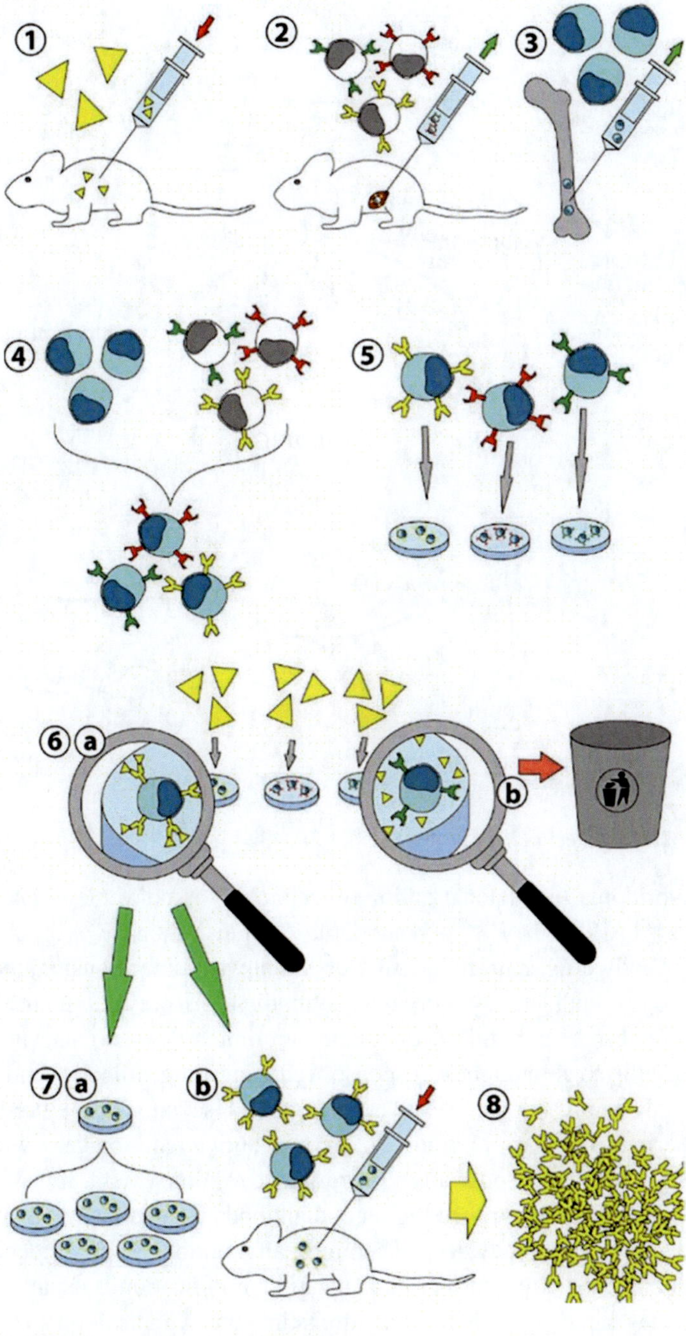

Figure 1. Hybridoma technology flow chart.

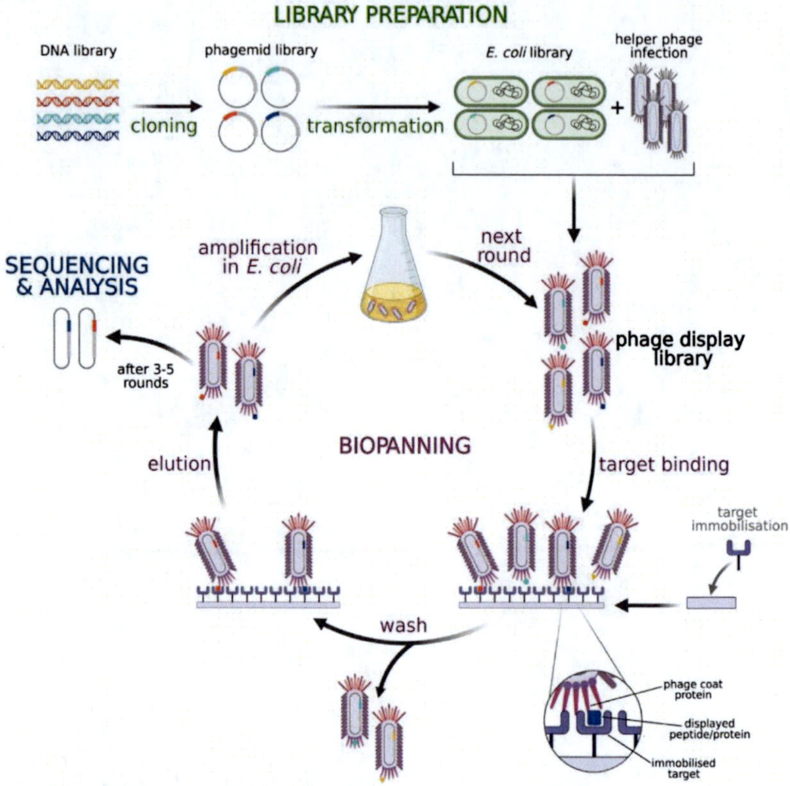

Figure 2. Phage technology process [18].

Hybridoma monoclonal antibody technology is convenient, simple, and low-cost. In 1986, the US Food and Drug Administration (FDA) approved the first antibody drug, muromomab-CD3, which was screened using hybridoma technology with mouse-derived antibodies. However, mouse-derived antibodies can be recognized by the human immune system, causing a solid human anti-mouse antibody response, reducing drug efficacy, and causing severe adverse reactions. To solve this problem, scientists have used genetic engineering methods to humanize mouse-derived antibodies, which has reduced human anti-mouse antibody response to some extent. It was not until 1994 that the FDA approved the second antibody drug, abciximab, a human-mouse chimeric antibody drug. Therefore, after antibodies are screened using hybridoma technology, further humanization modification is usually required before they can be used as antibody drugs in clinical applications.

Phage Display Technology

Antibody library display technology has rapidly developed over the past 30 years, becoming a leading tool in antibody engineering. Several display platforms have been introduced to produce monoclonal antibodies, such as yeast surface display, ribosome display, and phage display. As phage display is relatively more widely used compared to other display platforms, this section will provide an overview of this technology.

Phage display was first introduced by Smith in 1985 and further developed by other scientists. This technology is based on gene engineering bacteriophages (viruses that infect bacteria such as E. coli) encoding antibody (or other protein) genes fused with the coat protein gene of filamentous phages, with the products of these fused genes being inserted into the phage particle and expressed on the surface of the phage. In this way, a physical link is established between phenotype and genotype. Positive clones can be screened from the phage display library using fixed antigens, and the selected phages can be passaged, amplified, and further selected for several rounds in their bacterial host. Notably, the sequence of the displayed antibody can be obtained by determining the encoded DNA sequence packaged in the phage particles [14]. Researchers have used peripheral blood mononuclear cells (PBMCs) from immunized or infected animals or humans to extract total RNA, reverse-transcribe it into cDNA, and amplify the complete set of antibody heavy chain variable region (VH) and light chain variable region (VL) genes using specific primers to generate a large-capacity antibody library. The antibody library is then cloned into the gene encoding phage coat proteins for expression. Specifically, the library is electrotransferred into susceptible cells and assisted with phage transduction, and the supernatant collected is the phage display library [15, 16]. Antigen-specific antibodies can be screened from the phage display antibody library using various strategies. Here are two standard methods: the first involves incubating the phage display library with antigens immobilized on 96-well microplates. The affinity effect generated by solid-phase surface-bound antigens can simultaneously select weakly binding ligands, which are commonly used for the selection of natural libraries. The second method involves incubation of the library with biotinylated antigen in solution. Subsequently, the captured phages are immobilized on streptavidin-coated 96-well microplates, and this method can be used to select high-affinity clones by adjusting the concentration of biotinylated antigen and is more suitable for the selection of affinity-improved clones. Antibody fragments displayed on phage coat proteins include Fabs (fragment antigen bindings) or single-chain antibodies (single-chain antibody fragment, scFv). While Fabs are relatively stable in structure and have binding capacities similar to intact IgG antibodies, scFvs have weak immunogenicity, rapid clearance, and low molecular weight. Still, they are prone to self-reactivity or loss of binding affinity [17].

Phage display technology is not limited by animal immune tolerance. It allows the identification of antibodies against poorly antigenic antigens or those that are difficult to obtain using animal immunization methods. Technology only requires the gene sequence of the immunoglobulin, establishing a phage antibody library to screen for specific antibodies against the target antigen, shortening the experimental cycle and increasing stability. As of 2020, the US Food and Drug Administration (FDA) approved nine human antibody drugs produced through phage display to treat human diseases [18].

B Cell Cloning and Amplification Technique

With the advancements in immunology and technological development, direct screening of antibody-secreting B cells with antigen specificity has emerged as a novel approach [19]. Since natural B cells cannot be cultured long-term ex vivo, this method often relies on the differential expression of surface markers on plasma or memory B cells. Specific types of B cells are isolated using flow cytometry or magnetic bead selection, followed by short-term *in vitro* stimulation using cytokines to obtain B cell culture supernatant. B cells secreting the desired antibodies are identified through specific detection and their antibody genes are cloned for recombinant antibody expression. Alternatively, antigen-specific binding B cells can be directly cultured, or their genes can be retrieved by individually selecting B cells during flow cytometry. Antibodies obtained through these methods are naturally paired antibodies and do not require random recombination [19]. Compared to other techniques for monoclonal antibody production, the B cell cloning and amplification technique offers several advantages, including the preservation of naturally paired variable regions of the light and heavy chains, high genetic diversity, high efficiency, and minimal cell requirement. It is the most direct method for obtaining fully human monoclonal antibodies. This section provides a concise overview of identifying and isolating individual B cells, amplifying and cloning single-cell antibody genes, and *in vitro* stimulation culture of B cells.

Identification and Isolation Of Individual B Cells

Currently, the isolation and sorting of single cells remains a challenging technology, with the main challenges being whether the yield and quality (i.e., cell integrity and purity) can meet the technical requirements and whether the throughput and sensitivity of the single-cell separation method can meet the technical requirements. Some technologies have been developed successfully for single-cell isolation and sorting, which can be applied according to scientific objectives.

The isolation of individual B cells can be divided into random and antigen-specific isolation. The former only requires separating B cells, and the operation is simple. However, random isolation is suitable for blood samples with high concentrations of antigen-specific antibodies, usually from vaccine recipients or patients, to minimize the workload of subsequent antibody-specific identification. The latter requires the separation of antigen-specific B cells, which is more complex and particularly suitable for situations where the concentration of specific antibodies, such as anti-tumor antibodies and autoimmunity antibodies, is low [8, 20, 21].

The methods for random B cell isolation mainly include microscopic operation [8], laser capture microdissection [22], and fluorescence-activated cell sorting [23, 24]. Microscopic operation is the manual separation of B cells under the microscope. Although this method requires no special equipment, it has low separation efficiency and a limited number of separated cell types. The basic process of laser capture microdissection is to slice the specimen previously stained by tissue chemistry, immunohistochemistry, or immunofluorescence methods and observe the morphological and staining conditions of cells under a micro-laser cutting system to obtain a single-cell group or single cell. The characteristics of this method are simple operation, accurate positioning, and the ability to select the same type of cells and even single cells specifically from the sample and remove impurities. However, this technology has complex sample preparation and can only obtain a small number of single B cells automatically quickly. The fluorescence-activated cell sorting method is based on the fluorescent dye and cell sorter, using a laser beam to excite the fluorescent substance coupled to the antibody bound to the cell's single-flowing surface and automatically analyzing or sorting the cell based on the resulting fluorescent signal. Although the operation is more complex, and the equipment and sample requirements are higher, fluorescence-activated cell sorting can automate and accurately sort or analyze cells, making it one of the most widely used cell separation methods.

Antigen-selective sorting requires the effective screening and identification of B cells with the necessary specificity before IgG gene cloning, making the operation relatively complex. It is more suitable when blood samples contain low concentrations of specific antibodies such as autoimmunity and anti-tumor antibodies. Commonly used methods for this type of sorting include fluorescence-labeled antigen multi-parameter cell sorting [25], antigen-labeled magnetic bead sorting [26], micro-engraving, and cell microarray chips. Fluorescence-labeled antigen multi-parameter cell sorting is similar to fluorescence-activated cell sorting, with the difference that the former requires the addition of a fluorescent-labeled target antigen in addition to the fluorescence-labeled antibody used to label the B cell surface antigen to select the target antigen-specific Bcells. It can analyze tens of thousands of cells at high speed and simultaneously measure multiple parameters from a single cell. This technology improves the purity of separated cells, adds more cell information, and sorts B cells from different periods for different research directions. This has the advantages of high speed, high accuracy, and a high degree of automation and has become one of the most advanced cell quantitative analysis and sorting techniques. The fundamental principle of antigen-labeling magnetic bead sorting is based on the fact that cell surface target antigen-specific antibodies can bind to target antigens connected to magnetic beads in an external magnetic field and cells attached to target antigens and magnetic beads are absorbed and retained in magnetic fields. In contrast, cells without surface-specific antibodies that can bind to magnetic beads do not have magnetism and do not stay in a magnetic field, thereby separating cells. This method can separate high-purity cells from complex cell mixtures in a few and can be used for pre-separation before flow sorting single cells. Still, it is unfavorable for post-separation cultivation and operation due to the effect of magnetic beads on cell viability. Micro-engraving is based on the soft lithography microarray chip identifying B cells that can secrete antigen-specific antibodies, stimulating multiple cloning B cells to produce antibodies and placing them one by one in the chip hole. After the corresponding protein chip is transferred, a fluorescent-labeled target antigen can recognize the specific antibody, and the detected antigen-specific antibody B is transferred to a cell culture dish for subsequent clone operation. Like micro-engraving, the cell microarray chip method has high throughput, speed, cost, and ability to sort and identify antibody-secreting B cells from multiple clones directly.

System developed by Berkeley Lights in the United States, which can rapidly perform single-cell analysis through the integration of microfluidic nanoliter-scale micro-reactor technology, optoelectronic positioning technology, and computer systems, to the automation and integration of single-cell selection, cultivation, detection, and collection [27]. The antibody early discovery process based on the Beacon system can be summarized into five steps: immune and antibody secretion cell enrichment, antibody secretion cell plating, antibody cloning identification, positive clone screening and antibody sequence acquisition, cloning and expression. This technology has systematically innovated conventional methods, significantly shortened the development cycle, and improved development efficiency.

Cloning and Amplification of Antibody Genes from Single Cells

Obtaining specific antibodies through cloning and amplifying single-cell antibody genes involves directly lysing, getting antibody genes from sorted B cells, and then expressing and evaluating the antibodies after *in vitro* recombination. The advantage of this method is its speed and short cycle for obtaining antibody genes. However, the specificity of flow cytometry during antigen screening is highly required since only the binding to the labeled antigen during sorting is involved. Additionally, the screening of functional antibodies or antibodies requiring cell-based screening cannot be conducted in the initial screening phase but only after identifying and further screening antibodies capable of antigen binding in flow cytometry testing. Moreover, due to the low abundance of mRNA in single B cells, the specificity and sensitivity of bait gene primers and experimental operations are highly required [8].

During monoclonal antibody development, single-cell PCR technology amplifies target cells of circulating B lymphocytes in human or animal blood. B lymphocytes are activated and differentiate into antibody-secreting and memory B cells after antigen or lymphokine stimulation. There are advantages and disadvantages to using the two types of B cells to amplify antibody genes. Since specific memory B cells can be captured through antigens, this dramatically reduces the workload of subsequent screening processes. However, a large sample size is required. The low transcriptional content in memory B cells increases the difficulty of single-cell PCR amplification. Ody-secreting cells have a high separation rate, need less sample volume, and have a high PCR positivity rate. However, since non-specific antibody-secreting cells are still included, this increases the workload of subsequent screening. The discrimination between the two types of cells can be achieved by fluorescent labeling of different White cell differentiation antigen molecules on the cell surface.

Typically, appropriate primers are used to perform nested or semi-nested reverse transcription PCR for amplifying unknown antibody genes from single B cells. The primer design is crucial for achieving universal amplification with sensitivity and specificity that can avoid non-specific amplification and amplify complete antibody gene sequences. The forward primers are a mixture designed against different leader sequences of variable regions of heavy and light chains, while the reverse primers are specifically complementary to the constant regions of the antibodies. Depending on the experimental purpose, if different isotypes of antibodies need to be isolated and amplified, the reverse primers will be a mixture of specific complementary sequences of constant regions of all isotypes. In addition, to facilitate overlap extension PCR recombination and enzymatic digestion, the forward primers of antibody heavy and light chain variable regions need to contain restriction endonuclease recognition sites at the 5' end. In comparison, the reverse primers must include these sites at the 3' end. Although this method has been proven to amplify some antibody sequences, the diversity of products is still limited by the non-conserved binding sequences of the forward primers, which theoretically cannot cover all functional antibody genes among sorted B cells. Additionally, this complex multiple PCR reaction system based on mixed primers may have problems with amplification efficiency, specificity, and the restoration of antibody gene expression profiles [28].

It has been reported that cDNA 5'RACE technology can amplify variable structural domain genes from single cells [29]. B cells are isolated from blood, and gene-specific primers are used to synthesize the first-strand cDNA from single cells. 16-fold excess dGTP is added in the synthesis of the first-strand cDNA for G-tailing, and the second-strand cDNA is synthesized using oligo (dC) adapters. Then, PCR amplification of the cDNA is performed using primers that anneal to the adapter sequence and gene-specific primers. A nested primer is used for the second PCR, amplifying cDNA fragments that contain the complete variable region, including 50 untranslated regions, the leader sequence, and the start codon. This technique requires minimal materials, as small as a single cell and can amplify antibody genes that forward primer mix PCR methods cannot amplify. Moreover, no purification of PCR products is needed during the procedure, which eliminates the need for a complex mixture of forward primers and simplifies the reaction system.

The results of the amplified antibody gene products can be sequenced and evaluated for V-D-J gene integrity and analyzed for insertion, deletion, and mutation in corresponding databases, such as IMGT V-QUEST (http://www

imgt.org/IMGT_vquest/share/textes/) and IgBLAST (http://wwwncbinlm.nih.gov/igblast/).

***In Vitro* Stimulation and Culture of B Cells**

B cells in the blood are responsible for secreting specific antibodies, mainly consisting of memory B cells and plasma cells. Memory B cells are long-lived cells generated after antigen stimulation and can quickly proliferate and differentiate into plasma cells and produce antibodies when re-stimulated with antigens. Plasma cells, on the other hand, have a short lifespan in the body, usually only a few days. Therefore, it is crucial to stimulate and culture memory B cells *in vitro* to promote their proliferation and differentiation into antibody-secreting plasma cells to screen specific antibodies.

When memory B cells are re-stimulated with antigens, the CD40 ligand (CD40L) on the surface of Th cells is activated. It binds to the CD40 molecule on the surface of B cells, promoting the differentiation of memory B cells into plasma cells. In addition, many cytokines, such as IL-21, IL-2, IL-6, and IL-10, have been shown to act as co-stimulatory factors to promote plasma cell differentiation [30].

In a study, stable CD40L-expressing 293T cells were selected as feeder cells and co-cultured with human B cells using cytokines IL-21 and IL-2 for *in vitro* stimulation and culture. The feeder cells in the culture medium secrete CD40L, which can bind to the CD40 molecule on the surface of B cells, promoting the differentiation of memory B cells into plasma cells. In addition, cytokines such as IL-21 and IL-2 in the culture medium have been shown to act as co-stimulatory factors to promote the differentiation of memory B cells. The CD40L secreted by feeder cells mainly plays a role in stimulating B-cell differentiation. However, the mRNA in feeder cells can interfere with amplifying subsequent antibody genes. Therefore, feeder cells need to be irradiated with a sublethal dose before culture to ensure their inability to survive at the end of the culture. The number of feeder cells is also crucial for the *in vitro* culture of B cells. If there are too many feeder cells, they will compete with B cells in the early stages of culture, and if there are too few feeder cells, the stimulation effect will be insufficient. Flow cytometry sorting can cause unavoidable damage to cells and may lead to the failure of *in vitro* culture. An excessive number of cells can also cause difficulties in pairing the light and heavy chains of antibodies in later stages. Thus, minimizing the number of cells sorted per well is important while ensuring the success rate of culture. After successfully culturing B cells, the variable region genes of B cell antibodies can be retrieved and connected to the human antibody constant region to construct an antibody expression vector.

B cells *in vitro* stimulation culture is used for specific antibody screening. After isolating specific B cells, they are stimulated and differentiated in a particular culture medium to differentiate into antibody-secreting plasma cells. Then, antibodies in the culture supernatant are detected, and positive wells are selected for subsequent antibody gene retrieval. Compared to the single-cell PCR, antibody screening through *in vitro* culture provides more flexibility for selecting antibody specificity. The availability of 200 μL culture supernatant for detection facilitates functional screening of antibodies and cell-based in situ screening without waiting for screening and identification after recombinant antibody production. This increases the specificity of antibody screening and improves the likelihood of obtaining the desired antibodies [31]. Additionally, short-term culture (7-14 days) allows for the expansion of B cells, which partly reduces the difficulty of antibody gene retrieval (Figure 3).

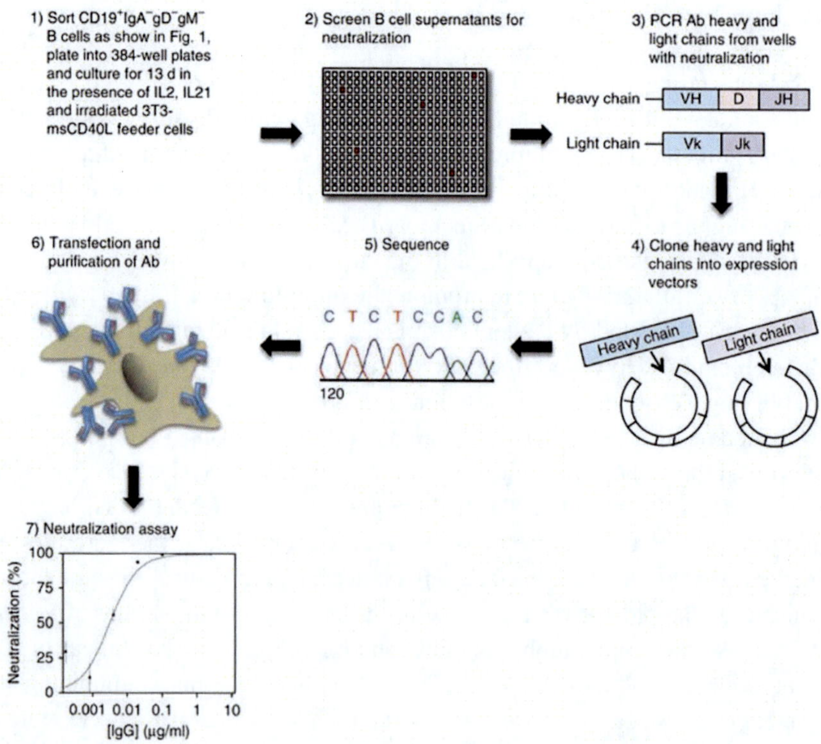

Figure 3. Workflow of human monoclonal antibody isolation [32].

Humanization of Antibodies

Since the establishment of monoclonal antibody (mAb) hybridoma technology in 1975, anti-CD3 mAb (OT3) was approved as the first therapeutic antibody in 1986 and despite high expectations for treating diseases using mAbs, OKT3, which is used for transplantation rejection treatment, failed due to the induction of severe human anti-mouse antibody (HAMA) reactions in patients. To reduce the immunogenicity of mAbs in humans, antibodies have been humanized using genetic engineering technology, yielding various forms of humanized antibodies. Since the 1990s, humanization techniques have been continuously updated and perfected. The current commonly used methods for producing humanized antibodies include framework-based humanization, species-based humanization, surface reengineering, and humanization based on complementarity-determining regions (CDRs). As the humanization of antibodies is necessary to reduce the HAMA effects of heterologous antibodies, this section will briefly review this technique.

Framework-based humanization involves CDR transplantation, in which non-human antibody CDRs are transplanted onto human frameworks [33]. Human frameworks with the highest homology to non-human antibody framework regions are typically selected as recipients for CDR transplantation. However, in more cases, direct transplantation of mouse antibody CDR loops onto human frameworks significantly reduces affinity. Humanized antibodies with species frameworks exhibit lower immunogenicity than humanized antibodies with IgG frameworks [34]. Humanized Fab fragments have moderate reductions in affinity compared to chimeric Fab fragments, and this form of humanization exhibits biological activity comparable to that of chimeric and hybrid Fab fragments and can display immune suppressive activity. Surface reengineering is another strategy for humanizing non-human antibodies, which involves replacing potential antigen surface framework residues with the most common human residues at positions that cause immunogenicity [35]. This method is based on human antibody responses to murine antibody variable regions being driven solely by surface residues. Humanized antibodies generated using this method typically exhibit little stability and affinity changes. The method based on CDR region homology is a new method for the humanization of antibodies, in which scientists hypothesize that mouse and human antibody frameworks with similar CDRs can support each other's CDR structures and retain the original antibody's high affinity [36]. In this method, human frameworks are selected without considering the homology of the framework regions, and critical mouse residues (hinge residues) are not restored in humanized antibodies. This method can reduce the possibility of being recognized as foreign and has been found to produce antibodies with good affinity while producing more antibodies than the framework-based humanization method.

Methods

Single B Cell Sorting

Peripheral blood mononuclear cells (PBMC) were isolated from convalescent COVID-19 patients' peripheral blood using a gradient centrifugation method [37, 38]. After antigen incubation and fluorescent staining, the cells were washed, filtered and made into single-cell suspensions for flow cytometry sorting. Memory B cells, undifferentiated B cells, and T cells were isolated and characterized by surface marker fluorescent antibody staining, and antigen-specific memory B cells were cultured by cell sorting.

B Cell Culture

3T3-CD40L feeder cells were cultured to a certain number, irradiated using an X-ray irradiator, and cryopreserved after irradiation. Irradiated cells and sorted memory B cells were mixed at a certain number and plated, allowing the memory B cells to grow and differentiate under conditions containing CD40L protein, IL-2, and IL-21.

Antibody Gene Amplification

Positive wells of specific B cells were lysed, and total RNA was released in each well. The first-strand cDNA was in each well, and V_H and V_L in the antibody were amplified by nested PCR. The first round of PCR was performed using a mixture of primers specific to the leader region and reverse primers specific to the corresponding IgH, IgK, or Igλ constant region or hinge region. The second round of PCR was performed using primers specific to FR1 and nested reverse primers specific to the corresponding IgH, IgK, or Igλ J gene or constant region. If the second round of PCR primers contained a restriction site, the product was sequenced and directly cloned. In addition, to avoid introducing AA by cloning using a primer mixture and the full-length lgk gene, the corresponding V and J genes were determined by sequencing the second PCR product. Then, another round of amplification was performed using V gene- and J gene-specific primers containing a restriction site, using the second-round PCR product as a template. All PCR products were sequenced before and after expression vector cloning. For recombinant antibody production, plasmids containing insert fragments with 100% identity to the original PCR products were co-transfected into HEK293 cells and antibodies were purified from the supernatant after culture.

ELISA Detection of Antibody Binding Activity

Enzyme-linked immunosorbent assay (ELISA) is one of the most commercially mature immune analysis methods, widely used in medical experiments, clinical diagnosis, and biopharmaceuticals [39]. Currently, there are four common types of ELISA: sandwich, direct, indirect, and competitive. Take sandwich ELISA as an example, a quantitative capture antibody is physically adsorbed to the surface of a microplate, the sample to be tested is added, labeled with a second antibody, and then colorized with TMB substrate. The color depth in the microplate positively correlated with the concentration of the analyte. Specific steps are as follows: coat a 96-well ELISA plate with fixed solution containing spike protein antigen of the novel coronavirus RBD to a concentration of 200 ng/well, add 100 μL per well, incubate at 4°C overnight; block: 5% skim milk/PBST, 100 μL /well, room temperature for 1 hour, wash with 1*PBST for 3 times, 300 μL/well (shaking at 500 rpm, 3 min); primary antibody: 100 μL/well of cell supernatant, incubate at 37°C for 1 hour, wash with 1*PBST 4 times, 300 μL/well (shaking at 500 rpm, 3 min/time), and positive and negative controls; secondary antibody: HRP-labeled goat anti-human IgG secondary antibody diluted in 1*PBS (1:2000) 100 μL/well, incubate at 37°C 1 hour. Wash with 1*PBST 5-6 times, 300 μL/well (shaking at 500 rpm, 3 min/time); colorization: add 50 μL TMB chromogenic solution per well and incubate at room temperature for 15 minutes. Add 50 μL 2M HCl to terminate the reaction, and detect OD value at 450nm. Statistical analysis: based on the experimental values, statistical analysis can be performed using software such as Excel to calculate the EC50 value of each experiment's antibody.

Antibody Affinity Detection - Bio-Layer Interferometry

Antibody affinity was determined using Bio-Layer Interferometry (BLI) on a Fortebio Octet [40]. Antibodies were immobilized onto seven anti-hIgG Fc capture biosensors at a 20 g/mL concentration. After establishing a baseline, biosensors were dipped into solutions of antigen at six different concentrations and HBS-EP buffer for binding and dissociation. (Kon) and dissociation (Koff) values were determined to calculate affinity (KD).

Microneutralization Assay

The microneutralization assay is an *in vitro* technique used to measure the capacity of virus-specific antibodies to neutralize virus infectivity [41]. Replication of the virus requires the supply of materials, energy, and replication sites from host cells, thus requiring active virus replication within host cells. After a virus enters the body, it attaches to the surface of a susceptible cell, penetrates and uncoats, invades the cell, replicates, and assembles the virus, thereby causing infection in the host. Specific anti-viral antibodies can inhibit one or more steps in the virus life-cycle after binding to the virus, preventing virus replication and infection in the host. In a microneutralization assay, the virus and antibody are mixed and incubated under appropriate conditions, the mixture is then inoculated into a sensitive host cell, and the remaining virus infectivity is measured. To perform the assay, antibodies were diluted 2-fold serially starting from 12.5 μg/mL, resulting in six different dilutions. SARS-CoV-2 virus and SARS-COV-2 mutant virus were diluted to 2000 TCID50. Fifty microliters of the virus were added to the gradient-diluted antibody, mixed, and incubated at 37°C for 2 hours. Cell suspensions at a density of 2×104 cells/well were seeded and inoculated with 100 μL/well of the virus-serum complex and then cultured at 37°C, 5%CO2 in an incubator. Cell morphologic changes (CPE) were observed after 96 hours, and serum samples that fully protected the cells were recorded for statistical analysis, which involves calculating the half-maximum neutralization concentration value (IC50) of each experiment's antibody using software such as Excel.

Animal Protection Experiment

The *in vivo* animal protection experiment mainly tests the prevention and treatment effect of purified virus-neutralizing antibodies against virus infection in virus susceptible animals. After the virus infects the animal, a series of symptoms appear, such as weight loss, raised hair, and death. Virus replication requires the provision of raw materials, energy, and replication sites from host cells, thus requiring active virus replication within host cells. By observing the symptoms and virus burden differences between animals treated with antibody therapy and negative control groups, it is possible to determine whether the neutralizing antibody can suppress the virus and protect infected hosts. Common experimental animals include mice, monkeys, and rabbits, and the dose and time of antibody administration can be set according to experimental requirements, typically less than or equal to 20 mg/kg, administered one day before virus infection (prophylactic experiment) or one day after virus infection (therapeutic experiment). If exploring the late therapeutic effect of antibodies, the administration time of antibodies can be delayed according to experimental requirements [42].

Specific Antibody Epitope Mapping

Antigens are molecules that stimulate the immune system to produce antibodies. An antigen epitope is a region on the antigen that an antibody can recognize; typically, an antigen has multiple epitopes. In contrast, a monoclonal antibody recognizes only one epitope on an antigen. Conformational epitopes comprise -15 discontinuous amino acid residues of primary structure brought together by protein folding. Antibody function depends on the epistatic interface created by the antibody and the antigen. Antibody function varies depending on the recognized epitope, such as activation or activity inhibition. Understanding the epitope recognized by an antibody is useful for evaluating the accuracy of antigen detection. Techniques such as competitive ELISA, flow cytometry, Western Blot, cryo-electron microscopy, and antigen-antibody complex crystallization can be used to identify the antigen epitope recognized by specific antibodies [43].

Virus Mechanism Identification

Antibodies are natural biological molecules produced by plasma cells or stimulated memory B cells in response to pathogen infection or vaccination. They are Y-shaped heterodimers composed of two 25 kDa light chains and two heavy chains of at least 50 kDa. Multiple disulfide bonds and non-covalent interactions connect the heavy and light chains. Antibodies can be divided into antigen-binding fragments (Fab) and crystallizable fragments (Fc). Two Fab regions bind and neutralize pathogens, while the Fc region connects to other effector molecules. Fab exhibits greater conformational flexibility than Fc and can strongly interact with antigens. Glycosylated Fc can bind to other proteins, mediating antibody-dependent cell-mediated cytotoxicity (ADCC), complement-dependent cytotoxicity (CDC), and antibody-dependent phagocytosis [44]. Fc can also interact with neonatal Fc receptor (FcRn), influencing the pharmacokinetics of antibodies. The sequence variations in different antibody subtypes determine their affinity and specificity for FcRn, FcγR, and complement protein C1q. IgG1 initiates ADCC and CDC, IgG2 and IgG4 are poor CDC activators, while IgG3 effectively activates CDC. Most clinically used or therapeutically developed monoclonal antibodies (mAbs) for infectious diseases are of the IgG1 subtype.

Antibodies can counteract viral infections through various mechanisms. Firstly, antibodies can prevent the binding of envelope viral glycoproteins or protein capsids of non-enveloped viruses to target host cells. These viral proteins have two main functions in the viral life cycle: binding to cell receptors and mediating viral-cell membrane fusion (in the case of enveloped viruses) or penetration into the cytoplasm (in the case of non-enveloped viruses). For example, the entry of SARS-CoV-2 into host cells is mediated by the interaction between the viral spike (S) glycoprotein and the angiotensin-converting enzyme 2 (ACE2) receptor on the surface of host cells. ACE2 is expressed in the respiratory, gastrointestinal, and endothelial cells. The interaction between viral spike and ACE2 can be blocked by antibodies targeting the receptor-binding domain (RBD), inhibiting viral infection. Antibodies that bind to complement protein C1q or FcγR on leukocytes can also counteract viral infections, leading to direct lysis of the virus and/or infected host cells. Antibodies can also promote or induce phagocytosis or the release of toxic substances such as cytokines or reactive oxygen species. In rare cases, suboptimal binding of antibodies to viral particles can facilitate viral pathogenesis through the antibody-dependent enhancement (ADE) process, where FcγR recognizes virus-antibody complexes and promotes viral entry into host immune cells [45].

Therefore, the ability of antibodies to neutralize viruses can be assessed through plaque reduction neutralization tests. The expression of intracellular luciferase can be detected to reflect pseudovirus infection, analyzing whether antibodies mediate ADE effects against corresponding strains. Anti-CD32 antibodies to block the interaction between the Fc segment of IG and FcyRII on target cells can be used to validate the occurrence of ADE effects dependent on the interaction between the IG Fc segment and FcyRII on target cell surfaces.

Conclusion

Monoclonal antibodies have emerged as critical scientific tools and powerful human therapies due to their high specificity for targets. They are increasingly important in diagnosing and treating malignant tumors, autoimmune diseases, and infectious diseases, with broad application prospects. So far, leading methods for generating, immunizing, and displaying therapeutic antibodies have been effective in producing antibodies against various targets and have received numerous commercial approvals. Hybridoma technology and phage display have provided essential approaches for isolating monoclonal antibodies, revolutionizing the field of antibody discovery. However, the low efficiency of the hybridoma isolation process and limitations of techniques based on prokaryotic expression have been critical technical limitations that take more work to overcome. Single-cell technology has advantages such as high efficiency, being fully human, and greater genetic diversity. However, the application potential of single B cell antibody preparation technology has not yet been fully realized, as it is constrained by practical conditions such as the inadequate development of high-throughput PCR antibody gene amplification technology, difficulties in preparing specific target antigens, and the demand for suitable human donors. Nonetheless, single B cell antibody preparation technology has become a popular method for generating human antibodies in the past decade.

Although some success has been achieved, the standard techniques for antibody discovery are time-consuming and complex. With an increasing number of antibodies entering the market, improving the antibody discovery process and creating more efficient technologies are necessary due to the limitations of current discovery platforms.

References

[1] Chon JH, Zarbis-Papastoitsis G. Advances in the production and downstream processing of antibodies. *N Biotechnol.* 2011;28(5):458-63.

[2] Haanen JB, Robert C. Immune Checkpoint Inhibitors. *Prog Tumor Res.* 2015;42:55-66.

[3] Blair HA. Ibalizumab: A Review in Multidrug-Resistant HIV-1 Infection. *Drugs.* 2020;80(2):189-96.

[4] Lee A. Ansuvimab: First Approval. *Drugs.* 2021;81(5):595-8.

[5] Posner J, Barrington P, Brier T, Datta-Mannan A. Monoclonal Antibodies: Past, Present and Future. *Handb Exp Pharmacol.* 2019;260:81-141.

[6] Weber J, Peng H, Rader C. From rabbit antibody repertoires to rabbit monoclonal antibodies. *Exp Mol Med.* 2017;49(3):e305.

[7] Buss NA, Henderson SJ, McFarlane M, Shenton JM, de Haan L. Monoclonal antibody therapeutics: history and future. *Curr Opin Pharmacol.* 2012;12(5):615-22.

[8] Tiller T, Meffre E, Yurasov S, Tsuiji M, Nussenzweig MC, Wardemann H. Efficient generation of monoclonal antibodies from single human B cells by single cell RT-PCR and expression vector cloning. *J Immunol Methods.* 2008;329(1-2):112-24.

[9] Liu JK. The history of monoclonal antibody development - Progress, remaining challenges and future innovations. *Ann Med Surg (Lond).* 2014;3(4):113-6.

[10] Holzlohner P, Hanack K. Generation of Murine Monoclonal Antibodies by Hybridoma Technology. *J Vis Exp.* 2017(119).

[11] Hanack K, Messerschmidt K, Listek M. Antibodies and Selection of Monoclonal Antibodies. Protein Targeting Compounds. *Advances in Experimental Medicine and Biology2016.* p. 11-22.

[12] Haupt S, Grutzner J, Thier MC, Kallweit T, Rath BH, Laufenberg I, et al. Automated selection and harvesting of pluripotent stem cell colonies. *Biotechnol Appl Biochem.* 2012;59(2):77-87.

[13] Nelep C, Eberhardt J. Automated rare single cell picking with the ALS cellcelector. *Cytometry A.* 2018;93(12):1267-70.

[14] Lu RM, Hwang YC, Liu IJ, Lee CC, Tsai HZ, Li HJ, et al. Development of therapeutic antibodies for the treatment of diseases. *J Biomed Sci.* 2020;27(1):1.

[15] Sheehan, J., and W. A. Marasco. *"Phage and Yeast Display." Microbiol Spectr* 3, no. 1 (Feb 2015): AID-0028-2014.

[16] Ma H, O'Kennedy R. Recombinant antibody fragment production. *Methods.* 2017;116:23-33.

[17] Lerner RA. Combinatorial antibody libraries: new advances, new immunological insights. *Nat Rev Immunol.* 2016;16(8):498-508.

[18] Jaroszewicz W, Morcinek-Orlowska J, Pierzynowska K, Gaffke L, Wegrzyn G. Phage display and other peptide display technologies. *FEMS Microbiol Rev.* 2022;46(2).

[19] Tiller T. Single B cell antibody technologies. *N Biotechnol.* 2011;28(5):453-7.

[20] Liao HX, Levesque MC, Nagel A, Dixon A, Zhang R, Walter E, et al. High-throughput isolation of immunoglobulin genes from single human B cells and expression as monoclonal antibodies. *J Virol Methods.* 2009;158(1-2):171-9.

[21] Menard L, Samuels J, Ng YS, Meffre E. Inflammation-independent defective early B cell tolerance checkpoints in rheumatoid arthritis. *Arthritis Rheum.* 2011;63(5):1237-45.

[22] Ogunniyi AO, Story CM, Papa E, Guillen E, Love JC. Screening individual hybridomas by microengraving to discover monoclonal antibodies. *Nat Protoc.* 2009;4(5):767-82.

[23] Jia B, McNeil LK, Dupont CD, Tsioris K, Barry RM, Scully IL, et al. Longitudinal multiparameter single-cell analysis of macaques immunized with pneumococcal protein-conjugated or unconjugated polysaccharide vaccines reveals distinct antigen specific memory B cell repertoires. *PLoS One.* 2017;12(9):e0183738.

[24] Shembekar N, Hu H, Eustace D, Merten CA. Single-Cell Droplet Microfluidic Screening for Antibodies Specifically Binding to Target Cells. *Cell Rep.* 2018;22(8): 2206-15.

[25] Starkie DO, Compson JE, Rapecki S, Lightwood DJ. Generation of Recombinant Monoclonal Antibodies from Immunised Mice and Rabbits via Flow Cytometry and Sorting of Antigen-Specific IgG+ Memory B Cells. *PLoS One.* 2016;11(3): e0152282.

[26] Jin A, Ozawa T, Tajiri K, Obata T, Kondo S, Kinoshita K, et al. A rapid and efficient single-cell manipulation method for screening antigen-specific antibody-secreting cells from human peripheral blood. *Nat Med.* 2009;15(9):1088-92.

[27] Winters A, McFadden K, Bergen J, Landas J, Berry KA, Gonzalez A, et al. Rapid single B cell antibody discovery using nanopens and structured light. *MAbs.* 2019;11(6):1025-35.

[28] Masri SA, Rast H, Hu WG, Nagata LP, Chau D, Jager S, et al. Cloning and expression in E. coli of a functional Fab fragment obtained from single human lymphocyte against anthrax toxin. *Mol Immunol.* 2007;44(8):2101-6.

[29] Ozawa T, Kishi H, Muraguchi A. Amplification and analysis of cDNA generated from a single cell by 5'-RACE: application to isolation of antibody heavy and light chain variable gene sequences from single B cells. *Biotechniques.* 2006;40(4):469-70, 72, 74 passim.

[30] Ettinger R, Sims GP, Fairhurst AM, Robbins R, da Silva YS, Spolski R, et al. IL-21 induces differentiation of human naive and memory B cells into antibody-secreting plasma cells. *J Immunol.* 2005;175(12):7867-79.

[31] Kwong PD, Mascola JR. Human antibodies that neutralize HIV-1: identification, structures, and B cell ontogenies. *Immunity.* 2012;37(3):412-25.

[32] Huang J, Doria-Rose NA, Longo NS, Laub L, Lin CL, Turk E, et al. Isolation of human monoclonal antibodies from peripheral blood B cells. *Nat Protoc.* 2013;8(10):1907-15.

[33] Cheung NK, Guo H, Hu J, Tassev DV, Cheung IY. Humanizing murine IgG3 anti-GD2 antibody m3F8 substantially improves antibody-dependent cell-mediated cytotoxicity while retaining targeting *in vivo*. *Oncoimmunology.* 2012;1(4):477-86.

[34] Pelat T, Bedouelle H, Rees AR, Crennell SJ, Lefranc MP, Thullier P. Germline humanization of a non-human primate antibody that neutralizes the anthrax toxin, by *in vitro* and in silico engineering. *J Mol Biol.* 2008;384(5):1400-7.

[35] Staelens S, Desmet J, Ngo TH, Vauterin S, Pareyn I, Barbeaux P, et al. Humanization by variable domain resurfacing and grafting on a human IgG4, using a new approach for determination of non-human like surface accessible framework residues based on homology modelling of variable domains. *Mol Immunol.* 2006;43(8):1243-57.

[36] Li PC, Liao MY, Cheng PC, Liang JJ, Liu IJ, Chiu CY, et al. Development of a humanized antibody with high therapeutic potential against dengue virus type 2. *PLoS Negl Trop Dis.* 2012;6(5):e1636.

[37] Gilbert AE, Karagiannis P, Dodev T, Koers A, Lacy K, Josephs DH, et al. Monitoring the systemic human memory B cell compartment of melanoma patients for anti-tumor IgG antibodies. *PLoS One.* 2011;6(4):e19330.

[38] Smith K, Garman L, Wrammert J, Zheng NY, Capra JD, Ahmed R, et al. Rapid generation of fully human monoclonal antibodies specific to a vaccinating antigen. *Nat Protoc.* 2009;4(3):372-84.

[39] Di Niro R, Mesin L, Raki M, Zheng NY, Lund-Johansen F, Lundin KE, et al. Rapid generation of rotavirus-specific human monoclonal antibodies from small-intestinal mucosa. *J Immunol.* 2010;185(9):5377-83.

[40] Li J, Schantz A, Schwegler M, Shankar G. Detection of low-affinity anti-drug antibodies and improved drug tolerance in immunogenicity testing by Octet((R)) biolayer interferometry. *J Pharm Biomed Anal.* 2011;54(2):286-94.

[41] Wrammert J, Koutsonanos D, Li GM, Edupuganti S, Sui J, Morrissey M, et al. Broadly cross-reactive antibodies dominate the human B cell response against 2009 pandemic H1N1 influenza virus infection. *J Exp Med.* 2011;208(1):181-93.

[42] Cao Y, Su B, Guo X, Sun W, Deng Y, Bao L, et al. Potent Neutralizing Antibodies against SARS-CoV-2 Identified by High-Throughput Single-Cell Sequencing of Convalescent Patients' B Cells. *Cell.* 2020;182(1):73-84 e16.

[43] DeKosky BJ, Lungu OI, Park D, Johnson EL, Charab W, Chrysostomou C, et al. Large-scale sequence and structural comparisons of human naive and antigen-experienced antibody repertoires. *Proc Natl Acad Sci U S A.* 2016;113(19):E2636-45.

[44] Schafer A, Muecksch F, Lorenzi JCC, Leist SR, Cipolla M, Bournazos S, et al. Antibody potency, effector function, and combinations in protection and therapy for SARS-CoV-2 infection *in vivo*. *J Exp Med.* 2021;218(3).

[45] Bournazos S, Gupta A, Ravetch JV. The role of IgG Fc receptors in antibody-dependent enhancement. *Nat Rev Immunol.* 2020;20(10):633-43.

Chapter 2

Delivery and Therapeutic Application of Neutralizing Antibodies

Qi Li[1]
Haonan Xing[2,*]
Aiping Zheng[2]
Yuanyu Huang[1]
and Mei Lu[1,†]

[1]Advanced Research Institute of Multidisciplinary Science, School of Life Science, School of Medical Technology, Key Laboratory of Molecular Medicine and Biotherapy, Key Laboratory of Medical Molecule Science and Pharmaceutics Engineering, Beijing Institute of Technology, Zhongguancun, Beijing, China
[2]State Key Laboratory of Toxicology and Medical Countermeasures, Beijing Institute of Pharmacology and Toxicology, Beijing, China.

Abstract

Neutralizing antibodies (NAbs) have been extensively employed as promising prophylactic and therapeutic reagents for preventing or treating infections, cancers, and inflammation-related diseases. However, their effectiveness is generally limited by short half-life, poor biodistribution, low bioavailability, and potential immunogenicity. To address these challenges, developing delivery systems to enhance biocompatibility, reduce swift immune clearance in vivo, and enable effective and targeted delivery of NAbs is critical. Herein, we provide an overview of the state-of-the-art achievements in the delivery strategies and therapeutic application of NAbs. First, a brief description of the

* Corresponding Author's Email: xinghn010@foxmail.com.
† Corresponding Author's Email: lumei@bit.edu.cn.

In: Neutralizing Antibodies and their Role in Health and Disease
Editors: Chenguang Shen, Yang Yang and Minghui Yang
ISBN: 979-8-89113-541-3

mechanism of action and classification of NAbs is provided. Next, we highlight the examination of literature pertinent to the delivery platforms, routes of administration, and therapeutic applications of NAbs. We hope this review can provide valuable insights for designing next-generation NAbs that integrate precise delivery strategies and administration routes tailored to specific therapeutic needs.

Keywords: neutralizing antibodies, delivery vectors, therapeutic application, administration routes

Introduction

With the emergence of the COVID-19 pandemic, NAbs have garnered significant attention due to their potential therapeutic applications. These antibodies protect host cells from pathogens by neutralizing or inhibiting their biological activity [1-2]. In 1890, Emil von Behring discovered antibodies in the blood of animals exposed to diphtheria or tetanus toxin and used them as a protective antitoxin drug [3]. The development of recombinant DNA technology in the 1980s enabled large-scale production and engineering of NAbs, which led to extensive research on their applications. In recent years, with advancements in our understanding of pathogens and the immune system, more NAbs have been discovered and utilized to treat various infectious diseases, including HIV, Ebola virus, and coronaviruses [4]. The global impact of COVID-19 has further emphasized the importance of research on NAbs and their therapeutic application. Several clinical trials have demonstrated their therapeutic potential against COVID-19 [5].

Compared to traditional vaccination, NAbs are used as drugs through passive immunization, thus offering rapid therapeutic and preventive effects. For example, certain chronic severe infectious diseases, such as hepatitis C virus and HIV, can be effectively inhibited by their NAbs. These NAbs have shown rapid and potent therapeutic effects against specific viral strains, surpassing the efficacy of traditional antiretroviral therapies in preventing infections [6-7]. However, the full potential of broad-spectrum, potent NAb vaccines for combating these diseases is still under active investigation [8-9]. In addition, NAbs have a shorter development cycle and timeline and may provide advantages during short-duration outbreaks, as demonstrated during the COVID-19 pandemic [5].

Despite the numerous advantages of NAbs, their short biological half-life following passive transfer poses a threat to maintaining therapeutic dosing, which necessitates repeated infusions. Non-specific endocytosis and proteolysis in body tissues and plasma and receptor-mediated phagocytosis by mononuclear phagocytes pose significant challenges to the efficacy of NAbs. Additionally, tissue hematotoxicity, low concentration at target sites, and biological barriers hinder the development of NAbs [10-12]. Therefore, searching for safe and effective delivery approaches is crucial for the widespread application of NAbs. Some commonly used delivery vehicles for NAbs include adeno-associated viruses (AAV), liposomal nanoparticles, exosomes, and B cells. AAV and various nanoparticle vectors significantly extend the half-life of NAbs [13-14]. As a delivery vector of NAbs, exosomes offer favorable stability *in vivo*, low immunogenicity, high biocompatibility, intrinsic targeting capacity and the ability to traverse biological barriers [15-16]. While B cell delivery platforms are still in the early stages of research, their high extraction efficiency, low immune toxicity, and high biocompatibility hold promise as delivery vectors of NAbs [17].

In addition to delivery vehicles, the choice of proper administration route also significantly impacts the targeting, bioavailability and effectiveness of NAbs. Intravenous injection can bypass the first-pass metabolism of the liver, allowing NAbs to be rapidly and efficiently delivered to the target organs and tissues through the bloodstream. Intramuscular injection of NAbs or their gene enables continuous production of NAbs and prolonged neutralizing effects [18-19]. Nasal administration and transoral nebulized inhalation delivery are easy and non-irritating administration. The two routes directly target the lungs without crossing the pulmonary vascular barrier, thus facilitating the localized release of NAbs for effective neutralization [20]. Intrathecal delivery allows brain-targeted delivery of NAbs by crossing the blood-brain barrier (BBB) through the cerebrospinal fluid [21]. Subcutaneous injection offers a convenient method with low toxicity, allowing gradual absorption of NAbs into circulation through lymphatic drainage [10]. Lens injection allows for the targeted delivery of NAbs by overcoming the ocular surface barrier [22]. So far, NAbs have been harnessed for therapeutic application in various fields and have yielded significant outcomes. Owing to potent neutralization, specificity, synergism, and therapeutic applications, a predominant application of NAbs is to fight viral infections, such as HIV, Ebola, Chikungunya, and Coronavirus [4]. In recent years, NAbs are increasingly being utilized in fighting bacterial infections, cancer treatment, and inflammatory diseases [10]. In this chapter, we provide an overview of the delivery and therapeutic application of NAbs with emphasis on the delivery platforms, routes of administration, and therapeutic applications, aiming at providing valuable insights for developing NAbs.

Mechanism of Action and Classification of NAbs

The neutralizing antibody (NAb) is a specific type that primarily binds to pathogens or other pathological factors, thus preventing the invasion of pathogens and reducing potential damage to host tissues. It is also a critical component of licensed antiviral vaccines. NAbs typically achieve their neutralizing effects by binding to antigens on the surface of pathogens, thereby blocking the interaction of the pathogen with host cells and alleviating or inhibiting the pathological effects on the host [23-24].

Mechanism of Action of NAbs

The mechanisms of action of NAbs can be divided into the following four parts, as shown in Figure 1.

1) *Blocking*: NAbs utilize neutralization property to attenuate or inhibit the pathogenic function of target molecules. By binding to specific receptors on the cell surface, NAbs block signal transduction pathways. NAbs will suppress the proliferation of tumor cells, which ultimately induces cell apoptosis [25].
2) *Anti-body-dependent cell-mediated cytotoxicity (ADCC)*: NK cells are innate lymphocytes with the remarkable ability to efficiently eliminate stressed cells, including virus-infected or tumor-transformed cells. The ADCC effect primarily relies on the activation of NK cells through FCR antibody binding and leading to the upregulation of CD16a expression. Upon recognition of IgG-opsonized targets via CD16a, NK cells unleash a repertoire of cytotoxic molecules that trigger the demise of the target cells. This intricate mechanism hinges upon the formation of immunological synapses and the degranulation of lytic granules containing perforin and granzymes. In addition to degranulation, NK cells can also engage target death receptors (such as DR4, DR5, or Fas) with their

corresponding ligands (such as FasL and TRAIL) to eliminate the target cells [26-27].

3) *Complement-dependent cytotoxicity (CDC):* Complement represents a group of heat-labile and enzymatically active proteins found in human or vertebrate serum and tissue fluid. The interaction between antibodies and complement C1 initiates a cascade of complement protein activation. It produced membrane attack complexes that dismantle the target cells and trigger the CDC effect. Numerous anti-tumor antibodies have demonstrated the ability to induce CDC, including those targeting CD20, CD52, CEA, and others [28].
4) *Cooperative interaction:* Antibodies can act as multifunctional carriers for drug delivery, combining with cytokines, toxins, or therapeutic agents to synergize their therapeutic effects. This strategy enables the localized and highly targeted delivery of cytotoxic drugs to tumor sites while conferring enhanced safety profiles on normal cells. For example, antibody-drug couplers rely on monoclonal antibodies that selectively bind to target cell surface antigens, facilitating their internalization and subsequent processing by the lysosomal system. This intracellular process enables effective drug release and leads to apoptosis. Moreover, a bystander-killing effect can further contribute to the death of apoptotic cells [25-29].

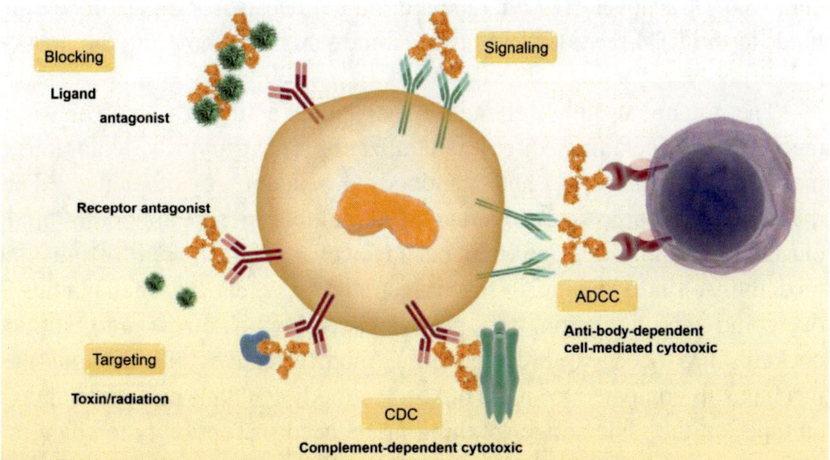

Figure 1. NAbs can exert neutralizing effects by binding to specific receptors and blocking the corresponding signaling. It can be used for therapeutic purposes through anti-antibody-dependent cell-mediated cytotoxicity, complement-dependent cytotoxicity or synergistic effects with cytotoxic factors.

Classification of NAbs

There are a variety of NAbs, according to different classification approaches. For example, NAbs can be classified as monoclonal and polyclonal antibodies based on their sources and preparation methods. They exert their effects through different mechanisms based on their structure and targeting characteristics. Polyclonal antibodies are less specific than monoclonal antibodies (mAbs). Currently, mAbs and antibody cocktails (monoclonal antibody conjugates) are more frequently studied. Besides, NAbs can be classified as monomers and multimers according to how the antibodies are linked and their arrangement. Depending on the number of binding sites, NAbs can be classified into monospecific and bispecific antibodies (Figure 2).

MAbs are produced from a single clone of antibody-producing cells, offering high specificity and consistency due to their single antigen binding site. They are pure and potent and exhibit remarkable specificity, making them valuable therapeutic agents for various diseases, including cancers, autoimmune disorders, infectious diseases, and transplant rejection [30-31]. For example, the chimeric mAbs c7E3 was derived from human-mouse hybrids. It explicitly targets integrin αIIbβ3 and prevents fibrinogen binding to vascular hemophilia factors, thus serving as an anti-platelet therapy [31]. Another notable example is ibalizumab, which is a monoclonal antibody approved as a novel HIV therapeutic after a decade-long gap. Ibalizumab binds to the CD4 receptor and prevents the virus from entering the host cell [32-33].

The immune response elicited by polyclonal antibodies involves various mechanisms, including direct neutralization, phagocytosis, complement-mediated destruction, and antibody-dependent cytotoxicity. These mechanisms synergistically operate when multiple specific antibodies bind to clusters of antigenic determinants. However, the limited affinity and bioactivity of individual mAb strains restrict their potential as therapeutics. To overcome this limitation, the precise assembly of mAbs into antibody cocktails has been explored, enabling more effective utilization of these mechanisms compared to single mAbs. Antibody cocktails recognize multiple epitopes on the same antigen, exhibiting reduced susceptibility to changes in antigen conformation. Experimental studies have demonstrated that cocktails comprising multiple mAbs show enhanced potency against viruses compared to individual mAbs. For example, the spike protein of SARS-CoV-2 is a critical target in COVID-19, and it has the potential to generate escape mutants with different phenotypes rapidly and become resistant under the selective pressure of host antibodies [34]. Studies have demonstrated that the prevalence of SARS-CoV-2 escape mutants can increase up to 10% in individuals receiving high doses of balanitis monotherapy [35]. The therapeutic efficacy of mAb therapy is significantly compromised, whereas the use of mAb cocktails minimizes the risk of escape mutants and has significant therapeutic effects. An example of an effective cocktail is SA55+SA58 which comprises multiple non-competitive antibodies that specifically target the receptor binding domain (RBD) of SARS-CoV-2, resulting in broad neutralizing effects against various SARS-CoV-2 variants [36]. Antibody cocktails such as casirivimab/imdevimab and bamlanivimab/etesevimab have also been employed in the treatment of SARS-CoV-2, providing neutralizing effects against a range of SARS-CoV-2 variants. Furthermore, *in vitro* experiments have demonstrated that mAbs cocktail therapy significantly reduces the emergence of escape mutants compared to treatment with individual antibodies [34]. These findings underscore the potential of cocktail therapy to mitigate viral mutations and improve therapeutic outcomes. It is worth noting that antibody cocktail therapy has also emerged as a promising approach in cancer treatment [37]. In addition, NAbs are primarily found in the form of proteins and nucleic acid drugs in their delivery and application. For example, the CR3022 protein antibody is used to treat SARS-CoV-2. In contrast, the hIL-15 protein is synthesized in vivo using the adeno-associated virus (AAV) carrying the hIL-15 gene to exert an anticancer effect [38-39].

NAbs can also be categorized based on their polymerization form, distinguishing between monomers and multimers. Polymers are more common as dimers and pentamers. For instance, immunoglobulin G (IgG) is a monomer that can coat bacteria, disrupting their function and activating the complement system. It also serves as a passive immune barrier for newborns. Immunoglobulin A (IgA) is a typical dimeric antibody predominantly found in mucous membranes throughout the body. Its role involves neutralizing bacteria and viruses and provides protective effects. Immunoglobulin M (IgM) is a pentameric antibody that activates the iron complement pathway, recruits immune cells and can adsorb viruses [40-42].

Compared to mono-specific antibodies, multi-specific antibodies with two specific binding sites have the advantage of binding both tumor and immune cells, enhancing the killing ability of tumor cells and blocking two signaling pathways to further improve cell killing. Additionally, the two binding sites enhance the specificity of these antibodies and effectively avoid off-target toxicities. Bispecific antibodies also have the potential to retain the effectiveness of combination therapy while reducing its toxic side effects. For example, AK104 is a bispecific antibody targeting PD-1 and CTLA. It showed significantly lower toxicity than the combination of PD-1 and CTLA-4. This may be attributed to AK104's superior affinity for lymphocytes, resulting in a higher safety profile compared to other antibodies that only bind bivalently to lymphocytes at peripheral sites, leading to tetravalent binding [43].

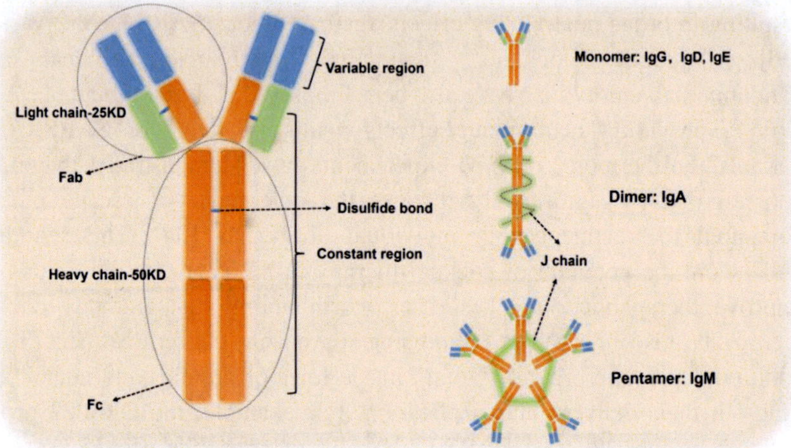

Figure 2. The typical structure of NAbs.

Delivery Platforms for Neutralizing NAbs

The relatively short half-life of NAbs in passive transfer necessitates frequent infusions to maintain optimal circulating titers. Clearance of NAbs by the immune system and the low concentration of NAbs at the site of disease reduce the bioavailability of NAbs. These inherent limitations have hindered the widespread utilization of passive transfer of NAbs as a viable approach for disease treatment and prevention [44]. Consequently, there is an urgent and compelling need for innovative delivery platforms to ensure more convenient and durable administration of NAbs. Such platforms would address the current challenges associated with passive transfer and significantly enhance the therapeutic potential of NAbs. These delivery platforms can be divided into adeno-associated viruses, liposomes, exosomes, and immune cells (Figure 3) (Table 1).

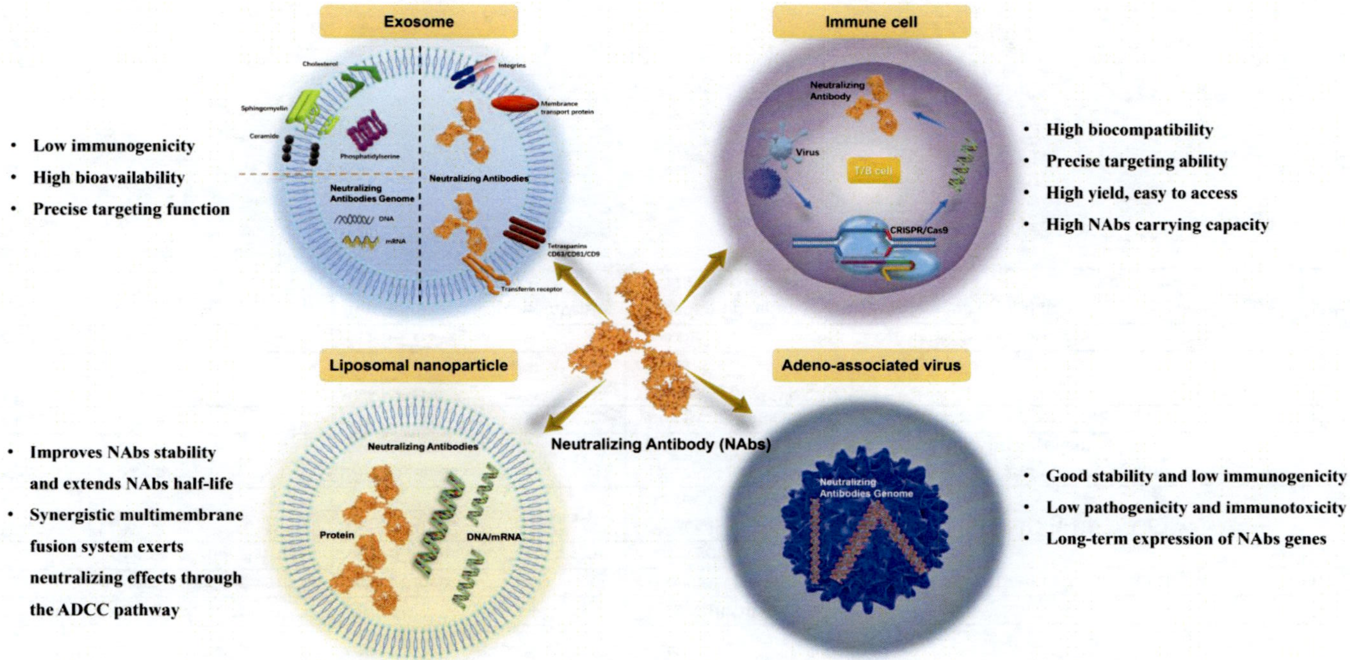

Figure 3. A summary of delivery platforms for NAbs.

Table 1. Delivery platforms for NAbs

Antibodies	Delivery platforms	Diseases or infections	Therapeutic outcomes	Ref
HIL15	Adeno-associated virus	Breast cancer	Efficient activation of LAK cell cytotoxicity for anti-cancer effects	[38]
IgG	Adeno-associated virus	Simian immunodeficiency virus	Reacts with (CDR)-H3 to treat SIV infection	[13]
HB27	Liposomes	SARS-CoV-2	LNP leads to longer circulating half-life of mRNA-HB27 and prevents SARS-CoV-2 infection	[14]
CHKV-24	Liposomes	Chikungunya virus	CHKV-24 mRNA inhibits viral replication and protects against arthritis, musculoskeletal tissue infection and lethality in mice	[51]
VRC01	Liposomes	HIV	Mice were protected from HIV attack	[52]
RBD-mRNA	Exosomes	SARS-CoV-2	Binding to the SARS-CoV-2 receptor binding domain exerts anti-infective effects	[15]
S proteins	Exosomes	SARS-CoV-2	Prolong half-life exerts anti-coronavirus infection function	[60]
CD20	T cell	Autoimmune encephalomyelitis	Targeting inflammatory cells within the central nervous system ameliorates autoimmune encephalomyelitis	[12]

Notes: LNK, lymphokine-activated killer; LNP, Lipid Nanoparticle.

Adeno-Associated Virus-Based Delivery Platforms for NAbs

Adeno-associated virus (AAV) is a non-enveloped virus of the genus Microviridae. It is a single-stranded DNA-deficient virus with an icosahedral and envelope-free microscopic structure. AAV has good stability, low immunogenicity, a broad host range, and long-expression of exogenous genes *in vivo* (Figure 4). Natural AAV variants serve as ideal vectors due to their inherent low pathogenicity and immunotoxicity characteristics. These properties contribute to high safety, enhanced stability, long-term gene expression capacity, the ability to accommodate a genome of approximately 5 kb, expedited expression kinetics, and the potential for engineering and optimizing viral capsids to further enhance the delivery characteristic of vectors [18, 45-47]. AAV as a delivery platform for NAbs primarily involves the transfer of antibody genes mediated by AAV into host cells and resulting in the production of endogenous antibodies and subsequent development of protective immunity. Skeletal muscle is an advantageous target for AAV injection due to its accessibility and high transduction efficiency with various AAV types. Following injection, AAV-carrying antibody genes can persist in muscle cells as non-integrated circular fragments, allowing for continuous synthesis of NAbs over time. This AAV-based delivery approach overcomes the limitations posed by adaptive immunity and offers improved bioavailability compared to conventional passive transport methods for NAbs. Moreover, while the half-life of NAbs in traditional passive delivery is limited (approximately 6 days), the AAV-based delivery system enables stable NAbs synthesis over an extended duration. It achieves long-term efficacy with a single injection. However, it is crucial to acknowledge the immunogenicity of antibodies and the potential binding of antibodies to off-target host proteins as significant considerations for the AAV delivery platform. Given the prolonged expression of antibodies in the AAV-based system, identifying effective strategies to regulate antibody expression remains challenging [19] (Figure 4).

AAV serotypes 8 and 2 vectors have been extensively investigated in clinical trials. They exhibit prolonged expression in humans, minimal preexisting immunity, no autoimmune responses following initial immunization and exceptional targeting capabilities in muscle and liver tissues. Notably, a recombinant adeno-associated virus type 2 carrying the hIL 15 gene successfully expressed the biologically active hIL-15 protein, demonstrating anticancer effects by activating the cytotoxic activity of LAK cells *in vivo*. This intervention effectively suppressed cancer growth and induced cancer cell death in transgenic mice with SV40 T/t antigen-induced breast cancer [38]. Moreover, the successful delivery of NAbs against simian immunodeficiency virus (SIV) in monkeys using AAV1 highlights the potential application of AAV in primate models [13]. The application of AAV-mediated NAbs delivery has also progressed to human clinical trials. In one trial, participants received the intravenous infusion of AAV1 expressing PG9, and no severe adverse reactions were observed, confirming the safety of AAV delivery vectors. Although significant PG9 antibody signals were not detected in serum, the presence of substantial HIV-neutralizing activity indicates the efficacy of AAV-PG9 and is potentially attributed to the low detection limit. In another clinical trial, VRC07 concentrations comparable to the in vitro were found in the serum of all participants following intramuscular injection of AAV-VRC07. The highest concentrations of VRC07 were sustained throughout the subsequent 3-year follow-up period [17]. While further investigation is warranted to address deeper immune-related concerns, the clinical data strongly support the potential of AAV as a robust delivery platform for NAbs.

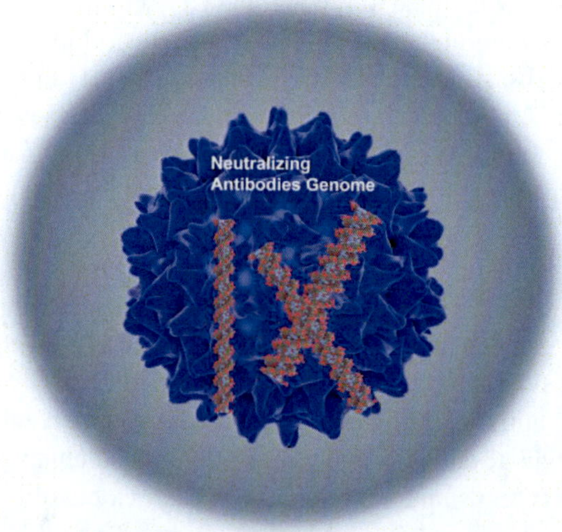

Figure 4. The structure of the adeno-associated virus.

Liposomal Nanoparticles as a Delivery Platform for NAbs

Liposomes are small vesicles composed of lipid bilayers that serve as effective carriers for delivering NAbs. From an electrochemical standpoint, most antibody amino acid residues undergo deprotonation and acquire negative charges. This property facilitates the encapsulation of antibody drugs within cationic liposomes, improving encapsulation efficiency and stability. Moreover, the surface charge of liposomes acts as an antioxidant, further enhancing the stability of NAbs. From a mechanical perspective, the hollow spherical structure of liposomes exhibits exceptional elasticity under pressure. Research has demonstrated a remarkably low coefficient of friction in aqueous solutions (as low as 2×10^{-5}) and a high maximum bearing pressure (up to 12 MPa). These characteristics ensure the stability and efficient circulation of NAbs delivered by liposomes. From a materials science viewpoint, liposomes, as nanovesicles, are formed by phospholipid bilayers that self-assemble through non-covalent interactions and this contributes to their superior biocompatibility [48-50]. Notably, lipid nanoparticles can be surface-modified and combined with other delivery systems to achieve reduced cytotoxicity and enhanced targeting capabilities. In conclusion, lipid nanoparticles can encapsulate NAbs effectively while improving their stability and bioavailability and prolonging their half-life (Figure 5).

For example, recent studies have utilized liposomes as carriers to develop a lipid nanoparticle-encapsulated mRNA platform for *in vivo* delivery of NAbs against SARS-CoV-2. This approach demonstrated the significantly prolonged *in vivo* half-life compared to conventional NAbs. A single prophylactic dose of lipid nanoparticle-encapsulated NAbs provided robust protection against SARS-CoV-2 infection in mice for up to 60 days, and the prophylactic effect exhibited a positive correlation with the dose of lipid nanoparticle-NAbs [14]. In a murine model, injection of lipid nanoparticles encapsulating mRNA encoding the chikungunya virus-NAbs resulted in adequate protection against arthritis and musculoskeletal tissue infection and led to nearly complete virus elimination within 24 hours of administration. *In vivo* experiments conducted in rhesus macaques further validated the potential of liposomal nanoparticles to enhance antibody concentrations and extend their half-lives, thereby demonstrating a dose-dependent therapeutic effect. These findings emphasize the efficacy of liposomal nanoparticles as a reliable delivery platform for NAbs [51]. However, it should be acknowledged that the delivery of lipid nanoparticles alone lacks immune escape and targeting functionalities. Cell membrane-liposome fusion systems have emerged as a promising approach to address this. Sun et al. proposed the ITHAP strategy which leverages platelets and liposomes to construct a bimodal fusion system for delivering lgG antibodies and cisplatin pre-drug aiming to achieve potent antitumor effects. This innovative strategy capitalizes on the precise targeting of tumor cells and immune evasion facilitated by platelet membranes. By employing membrane fusion liposomes, the stability and controlled expression of tumor cell surface antigen -IgG is achieved and leads to eliminating tumor cells with insufficient antigen expression via the ADCC pathway. *In vitro* experiments demonstrated increased NK cell adhesion and significantly higher NK cell abundance in the delivery strategy group compared to the control group. This affirms the adhesive properties of platelet membranes. The subsequent administration group exhibited notable tumor cytotoxicity (up to 47%), confirming NK cells' ability to induce ADCC. Furthermore, the robust bio-fluorescence distribution of tumors *in vivo* substantiated the targeting capability of the delivery system and the observed pathological changes in tumors underscored the therapeutic efficacy of this lipid nano-delivery system [11]. Furthermore, liposomal nanoparticles have been successfully employed as a delivery system for NAbs targeting various viruses including human immunodeficiency virus (HIV), rabies virus, influenza virus, Zika virus, and respiratory syncytial virus [52-55].

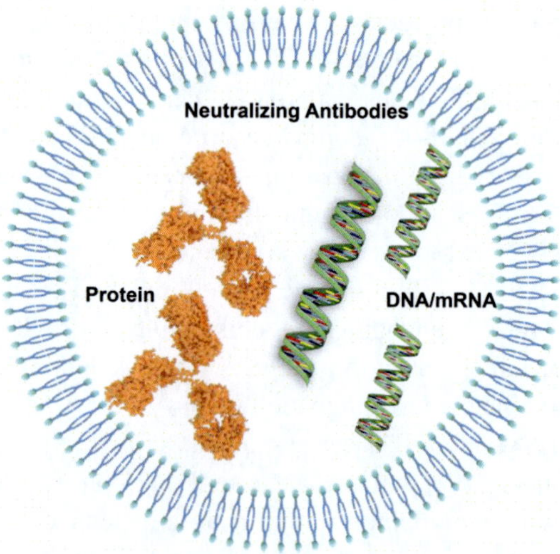

Figure 5. Liposomal nanoparticles as a platform for the delivery of NAbs.

Exosomes as a Delivery Platform for NAbs

Exosomes are nanoscale extracellular vesicles derived from cells. These vesicle-like structures have a typical diameter ranging from 50 to 150 nm and consist of lipid bilayer membranes. Exosomes play a crucial role in mediating intercellular communication by carrying proteins, DNA, and mRNA and serve as carriers for small molecule drugs or nucleic acids. Consequently, exosomes have emerged as promising natural delivery systems and are also used to deliver Nabs. Notably, exosomes exhibit low immunogenicity and high biocompatibility [56]. The surface of exosomes features specific "self-tagging proteins," including CD47 integrin which interacts with signaling regulatory protein α (SIRP-α). This interaction effectively inhibits their clearance by the immune system and leads to prolonged circulation and improved stability of the delivered drug [57]. Furthermore, exosomes derived from distinct cell types possess unique properties that enable them to overcome natural barriers (e.g., BBB) and exhibit targeting capabilities, such as inflammation or tumor targeting. For example, macrophage exosomes exploit the interaction between integrin lymphocyte function-associated antigen-1 and BBB intercellular adhesion molecule-1 to traverse the BBB [58]. Similarly, dendritic cell exosomes have demonstrated successful targeted delivery of siRNAs by specifically binding CD9 protein to receptor glycoprotein which assists it in bypassing the endocytosis pathway [59]. Regarding NAbs delivery, exosomes deliver corresponding binding proteins or RNA to induce the body to produce NAbs for further therapeutic effect (Figure 6).

A related study successfully developed exosomes containing the SARS-S protein, exhibiting promising immunological effects in the experimental mice. Comparative analysis with an adenoviral vector demonstrated that both exosomal and adenoviral vectors effectively generated NAbs and exhibited favorable therapeutic efficacy. Notably, the combined use of adenovirus and exosome vectors resulted in significantly higher titers of NAbs than those used alone observed in the sera of recovering SARS patients, indicating a highly effective treatment strategy for SARS coronavirus. In addition to their potential for protein delivery, exosomes can also serve as carriers for mRNA delivery. Zhang et al. utilized milk-derived exosomes to deliver mRNA encoding the SARS-CoV-2-RBD via inhalation. The experimental investigation *in vitro* aimed to assess the delivery efficiency of milk exosomes loaded with RBD mRNA into human cells. The results of protein blotting and ELISA analysis demonstrated that milk exosomes successfully delivered the mRNA into 293 cells. After 24 hours, the cells produced RBD peptides, which were secreted into the culture medium supernatant. Upon injection into the duodenum of BALB mice, sustained levels of NAbs were detected in the serum for up to 50 days, suggesting this delivery system's ability to elicit a prolonged immune response through inhalation. Furthermore, bacterial exosomes incorporating the SARS-CoV-2-RBD have demonstrated efficient delivery and extended the half-life of NAbs. It also reduced the viral levels in the lungs of a mice model effectively [15, 60-62].

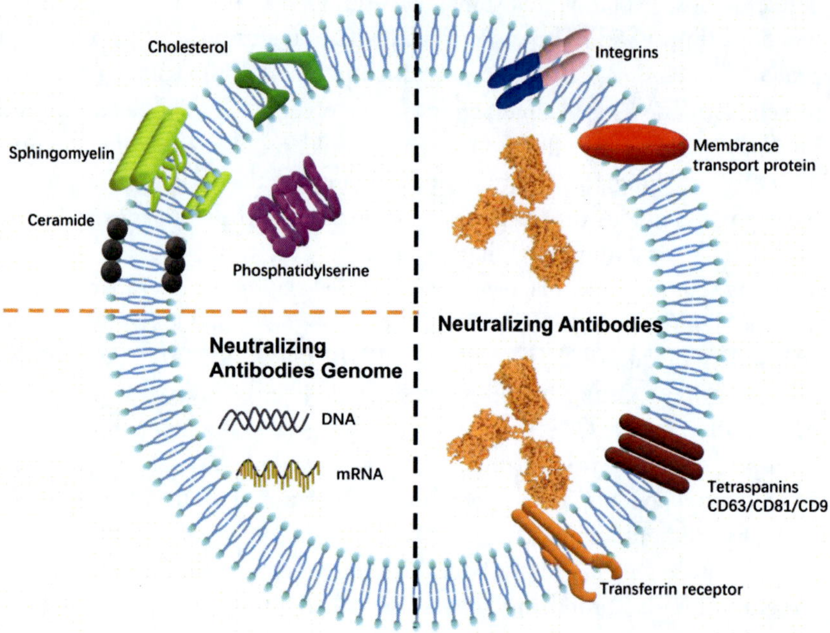

Figure 6. The structure of exosomes and the application of exosomes for delivery of NAbs.

Immune Cells as a Delivery Platform for NAbs

Immune cell-based delivery systems offer a biocompatible and precise targeting approach for delivering NAbs. Leveraging its inherent tissue and organ targeting abilities, NAbs can be effectively delivered to the specific lesion site. Compared to other delivery platforms, the immune cell delivery platform has the advantage of endogenous production and reduces the need for external preparation and complex purification. Additionally, immune cell carriers possess a large size and internal volume, allowing for a higher capacity to carry NAbs, thereby improving delivery efficiency and bioavailability. Immune cell delivery platform for NAbs can be achieved through direct external loading or modification of highly expressed NAbs. Among the immune cell delivery platforms, B cell and T cell delivery platforms are the most utilized platforms (Figure 7).

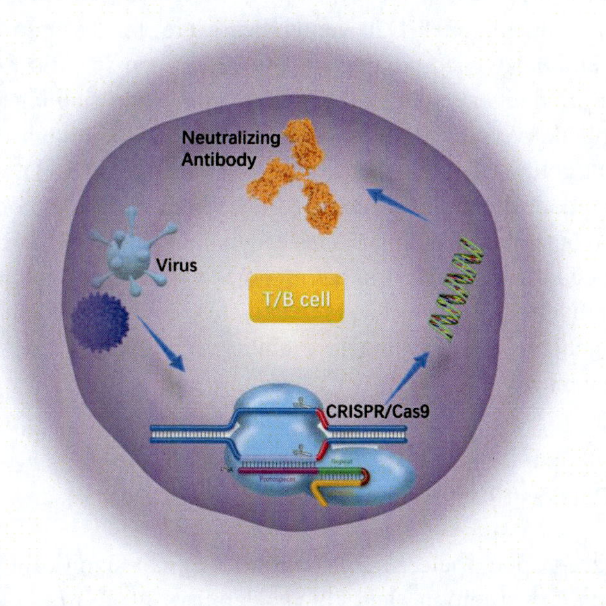

Figure 7. Immune cell-based delivery platforms for NAbs. The platforms are commonly designed by genetic engineering of immune cells using viral vectors and CRISPR-mediated gene editing for high expression of NAbs.

The genome of B cells can be genetically engineered using lentiviral vectors and CRISPR-mediated gene targeting to achieve high expression levels of NAbs [17]. In a pioneering study, lentiviral vectors were initially used to transduce B cells *in vivo*, resulting in the expression of the early Nab-b12. Subsequently, Fusil et al. reinfused the transduced B cells back into mice and observed a significant increase in the levels of hepatitis C virus-specific antibodies. Based on these findings, the advancement of gene editing technologies has led to the utilization of CRISPR-Cas9 editing to transduce proliferating B cells *in vitro*, leading to substantial production of recombinant protein [63-65]. Hartweger et al. successfully achieved robust expression of HIV-NAbs in both human and murine B cells using CRISPR-Cas9 gene editing techniques. Following the reinfusion of these modified B cells into mice, a notable increase in the concentration of NAbs was observed in the serum resulting in a potent neutralizing capacity [66]. In a recent study by Vamva et al., efficient expression of NAbs in human B cells was accomplished through a lentivirus-mediated B cell transduction strategy. *In vitro* experiments demonstrated the efficient ability of this protein to neutralize HIV [67]. As for the T cell delivery platform, Clara et al. created a T cell delivery platform wherein anti-CD20 antibodies were loaded into nanoparticles. Subsequently, they incorporated into myelin antigen-specific T cells, resulting in a bilayer delivery system for NAbs. Iron oxide staining confirmed the successful delivery of NAbs to the central nervous system (CNS) and the precise targeting of inflammatory cells within the CNS. The released anti-CD20 antibodies effectively depleted B cells in the spinal cord of mice and improved outcomes in autoimmune encephalomyelitis [12]. In conclusion, the immune cell delivery platform has emerged as an indispensable approach for NAb delivery. It is characterized by high biocompatibility, low immunogenicity, precise targeting ability, high yield, and high antibody-carrying capacity.

Administration Routes of NAbs

Selecting an appropriate administration route can significantly enhance the absorption, distribution and bioavailability of NAbs. An optimized administration route may ensure efficient drug delivery to target tissues and enhance therapeutic efficacy while minimizing potential adverse reactions. This section explores the various routes of administration for NAbs. Intravenous injection is the most common route due to its rapid onset of action, making it suitable for diseases that require immediate neutralizing effects. Intramuscular injection offers a straightforward and consistent delivery method, providing a continuous and stable release of NAbs. Nasal and oral inhalation are frequently employed for respiratory tract infections, as they allow for mucosal immunization and targeted delivery to the lungs. For example, NAbs-1212C2, administered via inhalation and specifically targeting the lungs to neutralize the SARS-CoV-2 virus, exerted antiviral effects [20]. Intrathecal injection bypasses the BBB by leveraging the diffusion of cerebrospinal fluid and enables precise delivery of NAbs to the brain. This approach has proven effective in neuropathic pain conditions where intrathecal administration of VEGFR-1 NAbs achieves desired outcomes [21]. Subcutaneous injection of NAbs offers ease of administration. With a slow absorption rate into the bloodstream through lymphatic drainage, subcutaneous injection provides long-lasting efficacy and convenient self-administration. However, it is limited to a single-dose administration. Lens administration directly crosses the ocular surface barrier, allowing for targeted delivery of NAbs to the intraocular region. This approach holds promise for treating ocular diseases that require localized treatment. Each route has unique advantages and challenges that impact the bioavailability, tissue targeting and therapeutic efficacy of NAbs. The selection of an appropriate administration route depends on factors such as the target disease, desired pharmacokinetics, and patient convenience (Figure 8) (Table 2).

Intravenous Administration

Intravenous administration is the predominant route for delivering NAbs. It enables rapid and efficient delivery of NAbs to target organs and tissues via the bloodstream and ensures high bioavailability by bypassing hepatic first-pass metabolism. This systemic approach is particularly valuable for diseases requiring widespread intervention. Intravenous administration is commonly employed in emergency and critical care settings to combat acute infections and life-threatening conditions.

Intravenous delivery of NAbs has demonstrated efficacy in various diseases. For example, the safety and antiviral activity of intravenously administered anti-HIV NAbs have been systematically evaluated, showcasing promising results against HIV-1. This is the first investigational report of a triple antibody combination for HIV-1 used in humans. Chien et al. demonstrated the effectiveness of intravenous administration of COVID-19 NAbs by verifying the dose and timeliness of the NAbs [68-69]. In an animal model, a high titer of B cell NAbs administered intravenously to rhesus monkeys completely protected the model animals from lymphocryptovirus infection. Lymphocytoma virus is primarily transmitted to uninfected hosts through oral secretions. It can bypass the oral epithelial mucosa to directly infect peripheral B cells, leading to the development of B cell and epithelial cell malignancies. Experimental data indicate that B cell NAbs provide protection against lymphocyte virus infection in rhesus monkeys, while epithelial cell NAbs do not exhibit the desired therapeutic effect. However, it is important to note that B cell NAbs may not confer protection in all animal models, and their antiviral effects might be attributed to the attenuation of acute viral load or sustained viral set point. These findings provide new evidence for developing NAbs via B cells [70]. Barouch et al. revealed the anti-HIV efficacy of PGT121 and 3BNC117 antibodies when intravenously administered to rhesus monkeys [71]. The experiments aimed to elucidate how

NAbs with incomplete neutralizing activity mediate protective effects *in vivo*. PGT121 exhibited 85% neutralization of HIV, while 3BNC117 demonstrated 70% neutralization; However, the inhibition of plasma viremia was dose-dependent for 3BNC117. These findings suggest that even NAbs with incomplete neutralizing activity can still exert antiviral effects and delay the progression of systemic infection which is crucial for virus prevention and treatment. Another approach is cocktail therapy, combining multiple strains of NAbs to address the limitations of individual NAbs. In conclusion, intravenous administration of NAbs has become the most widely utilized drug delivery route due to its rapid onset of action and other advantages. It has been employed in the treatment of various diseases. However, there are drawbacks associated with intravenous administration, such as increased consumption of resources, notable toxic side effects and the inability to achieve targeted drug delivery. For example, intravenous administration of bevacizumab can result in renal failure [72]. Therefore, selecting an appropriate drug delivery route should be based on individual circumstances and considerations.

Intramuscular Administration

Although vaccination plays a crucial role in preventing and treating infectious diseases. For individuals with compromised immune systems who cannot receive vaccines, intramuscular injection of NAbs offers a viable alternative. This administration route provides rapid protection independent of the immune system's condition, without relying on immune memory, and demonstrates significant efficacy in disease prevention and infection control [73]. Additionally, intramuscular injection of NAbs is a straightforward and convenient approach, offering comparable bioavailability to intravenous injection while bypassing hepatic first-pass metabolism. Skeletal muscle, with its accessibility, serves as an optimal site for intramuscular delivery, allowing temporary storage of NAbs or transduction of various NAbs genes. Notably, the NAbs genome can persist as stable non-integrated circular fragments within quiescent muscle cells and establish skeletal muscle as a reservoir for continuous production and release of stable NAbs [19]. Consequently, intramuscular injection provides a prolonged neutralizing effect compared to intravenous administration, as the antibodies are slowly released from the muscle tissue, allowing for sustained activity. However, its sustained effect makes it less suitable for emergency and critically ill patients requiring immediate treatment. It is worth noting that intravenous administration requires significant medical resources. Therefore, promoting the use of intramuscular injection as an alternative administration route for NAbs is of paramount importance.

A related study evaluated the efficacy of intramuscular injection of the Nab-AZD7442 for SARS-CoV-2 in adults with COVID-19. The results demonstrated that a 300 mg intramuscular injection of AZD7442 exhibited higher potency in achieving seronegativity against SARS-CoV-2 than recovery serum. Furthermore, even after 9 months, serum NAbs titers against SARS-CoV-2 remained three times higher than those associated with convalescent plasma, and the presence of AZD7442 antibodies was detected in the nasal mucosa [73]. It illustrates that intramuscular injection prolongs the neutralizing effect of NAbs. In addition to standalone NAb injections, intramuscular injection is well-suited for delivering NAbs gene vectors. For instance, an R1a-B6 nanoantibody designed to neutralize influenza binds to a highly conserved epitope in the HA stem, inhibiting virus membrane fusion. The target gene is packaged into AAV vectors through triple transfection, and intramuscular injection of AAV facilitates the efficient delivery of the NAbs gene to muscle cells by crossing the vascular barrier. *In vitro* neutralization experiments have demonstrated dose-dependent viral neutralization with the AAV genome, including cross-neutralization against influenza strains IA of H2, H5, and H9 [74]. Intramuscular immunoglobulin infusions in humans are primarily used for the prevention and treatment of specific infectious diseases, such as bacterial streptococci, Neisseria meningitides, diphtheria, and tetanus, and less frequently for immunodeficiency diseases [75-76]. In conclusion, intramuscular injection of NAbs has become an indispensable delivery route due to its adaptability to different conditions, and continuous and stable antibody production.

Nasal Administration

The conventional delivery method for NAbs mainly involves needle injection, which needs high doses and can lead to local inflammatory reactions, infections and other complications. Therefore, researchers have been actively exploring alternative delivery routes. Among them, mucosal delivery methods have gained significant attention, particularly the nasal mucosal route. The nasal mucosal immune route offers simplicity, cost-effectiveness, painlessness, non-irritation and non-invasiveness, making it highly suitable for patient use. Moreover, the nasal cavity exhibits minimal enzymatic activity, minimizing the risk of NAbs degradation. In respiratory viral infections, the adherence of the virus to the respiratory mucosa plays a pivotal role in the infection process. Nasal mucosal antibodies are crucial in capturing the virus, as they can impede virus movement and prevent further spread. Moreover, these antibodies exhibit a neutralizing effect, effectively neutralizing the virus and curtailing its dissemination. As a result, the virus and the antibodies are eliminated from the body through mucosal secretions. Thus, nasal mucosal delivery holds therapeutic potential and serves as a barrier against virus transmission, making it a valuable approach in combating respiratory viral infections [72]. Currently, most clinical administration of NAbs against respiratory viruses (e.g., SARA-CoV-2) is performed intravenously, resulting in suboptimal bioavailability in the lungs and limited therapeutic efficacy [77]. Patient management and adherence to intravenous infusion of specific NAbs is one of the factors contributing to the high cost and challenges associated with the treatment of novel coronaviruses. Therefore, intranasal administration has emerged as a promising route for delivering NAbs.

In an experiment by Halwe et al., a fully human monoclonal NAb called DZIF-10cto targets the RBD of the SARS-CoV-2 spike protein. It was intranasally administered to mice. The results demonstrated a significant reduction in lung viral particles and attenuated pathological changes during prophylactic treatment [78]. An et al. developed a novel IgM subtype antibody by assembling IgG and IgM antibodies. It was delivered to the lung mucous membranes through intranasal respiratory nebulization. The assembled antibodies exhibited enhanced neutralizing activity, blocking effect, and broad resistance to various new coronavirus mutants, effectively countering drug resistance from mutations. *In vivo* experiments in mice demonstrated that IgM subtype antibodies provided a wide range of protective effects both prophylactically and therapeutically [79]. Furthermore, several studies in animal models of the influenza A virus have shown that intranasal administration of NAbs is therapeutically superior to systemic administration [30-80-81]. Recent studies in mice have also demonstrated the efficacy of intranasal inhalation of NAbs against SARS-CoV-2. NAbs-1212C2 was derived from IgM memory B cells of COVID-19 patients and exhibits a specific affinity for SARS-CoV-2 spike proteins, demonstrating potent neutralization against the virus. Parenteral administration of MAbs-1212C2 has already demonstrated prophylactic and therapeutic efficacy. Subsequent administration of MAbs-1212C2 through inhalation further substantiated its viral neutralization effect by assessing body weights, pathological changes and viral titers in mice. Notably, the intranasal delivery of MAbs-1212C2 exhibited significantly higher administration efficiency, indicating enhanced bioavailability in target organs. The viral neutralization effect and administration efficiency of MAbs-1212C2 were markedly superior to those achieved through parenteral administration which underscores the enhanced bioavailability of this therapeutic agent in target organs when delivered intranasally [20]. In conclusion, intranasal administration represents a convenient and effective delivery route for NAbs, particularly in targeting the lungs. Compared to systemic administration, intranasal delivery offers ease of administration and improved bioavailability. Given the ongoing global prevalence of novel coronavirus pneumonia, intranasal administration holds significant potential as a valuable approach for effective NAbs delivery.

Transoral Nebulized Inhalation

Transoral nebulized pulmonary inhalation provides a convenient and non-invasive approach for administering NAbs. Converting the active ingredient into fine droplets can be inhaled through the mouth and delivered to the respiratory tract. This targeted delivery method enables the rapid and efficient delivery of high levels of NAbs to the respiratory tract, establishing mucosal immunity and effectively preventing viral infection and invasion at the mucosal surface of the respiratory tract. This non-invasive route is particularly valuable for respiratory diseases and offers a potent therapeutic strategy. Compared to systemic drug delivery methods such as intravenous or intramuscular administration, transoral nebulization bypasses the pulmonary vascular barrier. It allows for the rapidly accumulating high drug concentrations in the lungs and addresses limitations associated with drug distribution via systemic circulation. This approach improves drug availability, reduces costs and minimizes potential drug toxicity and side effects. Intranasal administration is another form of mucosal drug delivery that enables the uptake and penetration of NAbs across the nasal airway mucosa [82-83]. However, it is crucial to consider that this route of administration may lead to partial degradation of the administered antibodies and subsequently result in reduced bioavailability. Additionally, the nasal transmucosal uptake of antibody-antigen complexes can trigger antigen-presenting cells to process the complexes, thereby inducing immune responses within local lymphoid follicles [84]. Consequently, oral nebulized antibodies hold significant potential in achieving therapeutic efficacy in treating respiratory infectious diseases.

Ying et al. investigated the delivery of a bispecific antibody targeting SARS-CoV-2 via nebulized inhalation in mice, comparing it with intraperitoneal injection. The results revealed significantly higher antibody concentrations in the lungs of nebulized mice which demonstrated the direct organ targeting of nebulized inhalation. *In vivo* experiments showed that the nebulized bispecific antibodies effectively reduced lung virus titers. Moreover, *in vitro* assays of Vero E6 cells and mice lung homogenates demonstrated the bispecific antibodies' robust clearance of surviving viruses. There have also been studies of antibody-containing sera collected from patients recovering from COVID-19 to neutralize the virus entering the lung epithelium. A pulmonary nebulization system has therefore been proposed to prevent, treat, or immunize against COVID-19 infection [85-86]. Overall, the nebulized administration of NAbs holds substantial promise for treating various pulmonary diseases.

Intrathecal Administration

The incidence of brain diseases is increasing steadily. Yet, the presence of the BBB hinders the delivery of 97% of small-molecule drugs and all large-molecule therapeutic drugs to the brain for effective treatment [87]. Intrathecal injection involves injecting drugs directly into the subarachnoid space via lumbar puncture. It allows the drugs to diffuse across the BBB through the cerebrospinal fluid, rapidly reaching high concentrations in the brain. This administration route offers a promising approach for treating brain diseases, as it avoids the need for large-dose intravenous administration and reduces associated side effects. Moreover, it facilitates the elimination of necrotic brain tissues and bacteria by aiding the drainage of the diffused drug in the ventricles and mitigating arachnoid adhesion. However, intrathecal injection requires multiple doses to achieve therapeutic effects, posing challenges in patient compliance and the risk of bacterial infection [88]. Nevertheless, intrathecal injection remains a common and valuable administration route for brain-targeted drug delivery.

Meningeal metastasis refers to the spread of tumor cells to the meninges of the cerebral ventricles. This condition is characterized by a short survival cycle of approximately 3 months and is accompanied by severe clinical reactions. Conventional intravenous or oral medications have limited efficacy in reaching the brain and spinal cord due to the presence of the BBB. Thus, intrathecal delivery has emerged as a crucial method for delivering drugs across the BBB. In a study conducted by Glitza et al., it was observed that the immune cells of patients with advanced solid tumors, meningeal or spinal cord metastases expressing high levels of immunomodulatory molecules such as PD-1 and PD-L1 in the cerebrospinal fluid. These patients were treated with PD-1 antibodies using intrathecal administration. The results demonstrated favorable safety profiles, with only grade 1 adverse reactions reported. Notably, one out of 15 patients with advanced brain cancer experienced a significant remission of cerebral and spinal cord lesions with long-lasting efficacy. Additionally, four patients exhibited stable lesions and the median overall survival time reached 19.4 weeks. While the treatment effect may be limited, this study underscores the feasibility of intrathecal injection as a promising therapeutic modality for patients with advanced brain cancer [89]. Intrathecal injections of NAbs have also been explored for the treatment of neuropathic pain. VEGFR-1 is a neuroprotective molecule that can activate neuronal firing to produce neuropathic pain, and it also will be released in significantly increased amounts during chemotherapy, which contributes to chemotherapy-induced neuropathic pain. Researchers employed intrathecal injections of VEGFR-1 NAbs to achieve targeted analgesia. The expression of VEGFR-1 in astrocytes was assessed through fluorescence co-localization. Mice receiving intrathecal injections of NAbs demonstrated significantly higher thresholds to hot and cold stimuli than mice with neuropathic pain. These findings highlight the potential of intrathecal injection of NAbs as an efficient approach for the treatment of neuropathic pain [21]. Although intrathecal injection plays a pivotal role in brain-targeted drug delivery, careful consideration must be given to patient compliance and operational expertise.

Subcutaneous and Lens Administration

Subcutaneous administration involves delivering NAbs via injectable formulations into the subcutaneous tissues and providing localized and systemic therapeutic effects. Subcutaneous injection offers advantages, including reduced systemic side effects and sustained plasma concentration. Antibodies are predominantly absorbed at the injection site, minimizing direct entry into the circulation and reducing systemic toxicity. The slow and controlled release of antibodies from subcutaneous tissues maintains stable drug concentrations and ensures sustained therapeutic effects. Subcutaneous injection is distinguished by its dose flexibility, ease of administration, and potential for self-administration, which make it an indispensable route for delivering NAbs. Studies have demonstrated that the subcutaneous administration of NAbs targeting endothelial monocyte-activating protein II effectively inhibits lung endothelial cell apoptosis and inflammation and facilitates lung injury repair [90]. Subcutaneous immunoglobulin injections for primary immunodeficiency disorders have also demonstrated the therapeutic potential of subcutaneously administered NAbs [76-91-92].

In addition to the aforementioned routes of NAbs administration, ocular lens injection offers a distinct approach. Direct injection into the ocular lens enables precise targeting of ocular diseases by delivering NAbs directly to the affected area. This method circumvents systemic distribution and metabolism of the drug, providing a high concentration of therapeutic dosage to localized areas of ocular diseases while minimizing systemic toxicity and side effects. Additionally, it overcomes the eye surface barrier. Although ocular drug delivery is limited by the anatomical and physiological characteristics of the eye, lens injection facilitates the passage of NAbs across this barrier and enhances drug bioavailability within the eye. For instance, ranibizumab is an NAb used to treat wet age-related macular degeneration, and it is the first therapeutic agent approved for targeted ocular delivery [22].

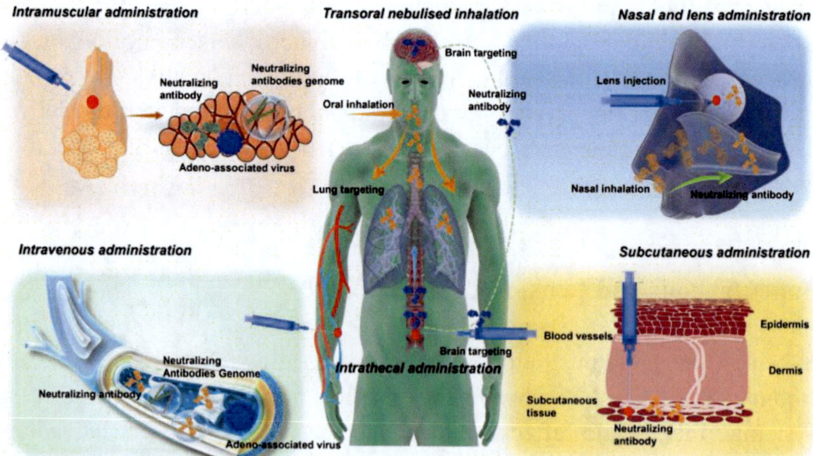

Figure 8. The administration routes of NAbs.

Table 2. Administration routes of NAbs

Antibodies	Administration routes	Diseases or infections	Therapeutic outcomes	Ref
PGDM1400	Intravenous administration	HIV	Reduction of HIV levels in plasma	[69]
PGT121	Intravenous administration	HIV	Reduction of HIV levels in plasma	[70]
R1a-B6	Intramuscular administration	Influenza virus	Binds to a highly conserved epitope in the HA stem and inhibits virus membrane fusion	[73]
DZIF-10	Nasal administration	COVID-19 Infection	Targeting the RBD of the SARS-CoV-2 spike protein reduces viral particles in the lungs and ameliorates pathologic changes	[78]
IgM subtype	Nasal administration	COVID-19 Infection	Blocking effect and broad resistance to various new coronavirus mutants	[79]
1212C2	Nasal administration	COVID-19 Infection	Binding to SARS-CoV-2 spike proteins for antiviral effects; Lung targeting	[20]
Bn03	Transoral nebulized inhalation	COVID-19 Infection	Effective removal of survival virus from lung cell	[86]
VEGFR-1	Intrathecal administration	Neuropathic pain	Crossing the BBB to inhibit neuronal activation and thereby reduce neuropathic pain	[21]
EMAPII	Subcutaneous administration	lung injury	Targeting endothelial monocyte activation protein II inhibits pulmonary endothelial cell apoptosis and lung inflammation	[90]
Ranibizumab	Len administration	Wet age-related macular degeneration	Crossing the ocular surface barrier for efficacy	[22]

Notes: HIV, human immunodeficiency virus; RBD, receptor binding domain.

Table 3. Therapeutic application of Nabs

Antibodies	Delivery platforms	Diseases and infections	Therapeutic outcomes	Ref
B12	AAV	HIV	Extend half-life and improved neutralization potency	[17]
Immunoadhesin	AAV	HIV	Block SIV active protein	[102]
3BNC60	B Cell	HIV	Reduce serum HIV concentration and increase neutralization efficacy	[66]
RBD-mRNA	Exosomes	SARS-CoV-2	Binding to the SARS-CoV-2 receptor binding domain exerts anti-infective effects	[15]
HB27	Liposomes	SARS-CoV-2	LNP leads to longer circulating half-life of mRNA-HB27 and prevents SARS-CoV-2 infection	[14]
HIL15	AAV	Breast cancer	Anti-cancer effects through activation of cytotoxicity of LAK cells	[38]
IN006	Nasal administration	SARS-CoV-2	Capture and neutralize virus-like particles in the respiratory mucosa	[113]
lgG	Subcutaneous administration	Antibody immunodeficiency	Reduce toxic side effects and compensate for immunodeficiency	[129]

Notes: AAV, adeno-associated virus; HIV, human immunodeficiency virus; SIV, simian immunodeficiency virus; LAK, lymphokine-activated killer.

Therapeutic Application of NAbs

The application of NAbs delivered by different vehicles to treat different diseases depends on the specificity of target tissues for specific therapeutic purposes. NAbs can specifically target key antigenic structures on the surface of pathogens and effectively block their ability to infect host cells. NAbs have demonstrated remarkable efficacy in combating viral and bacterial infections in infectious diseases. Moreover, their potential applications in cancer immunotherapy have garnered significant attention. Recent studies have also unveiled the potential of NAbs in addressing autoimmune diseases, rheumatoid arthritis and intestinal inflammation. The widespread utilization of NAbs presents new avenues for enhancing clinical care and propels further research and development of innovative therapeutic tools (Table 3).

Application of NAbs in Infectious Diseases

NAbs play a crucial role in combating viral infections by specifically binding to critical antigenic structures on the surface of viruses, thereby effectively blocking viral entry into host cells or inhibiting their replication process. Extensive research has demonstrated the therapeutic efficacy of NAbs against a wide range of viral infections, including HIV, Ebola, chikungunya, and coronaviruses. NAbs vectors also play a crucial role in the antivirus region [20, 30, 93]. Furthermore, the emergence of novel coronaviruses has led to the development of an increasing number of COVID-19 NAbs [86]. Highlighting their potential application in addressing emerging and critical viral infections. The development of NAbs and NAbs mucosal delivery thus offers new strategies and hope for antiviral therapy. In bacterial infections, NAbs also hold promise. They can prevent damage to host cells by binding and neutralizing bacterial toxins or inhibiting bacterial entry into host cells by binding to surface receptors. Furthermore, NAbs can modulate immune responses. For example, NAbs against Klebsiella pneumoniae have shown potential in attenuating the damage caused by its toxins to the respiratory mucosa. Additionally, antibodies targeting bacterial surface adhesion proteins have demonstrated the ability to inhibit bacterial invasion and adhesion [94]. In summary, the study and development of NAbs provide valuable avenues for antiviral and antibacterial treatments and present novel strategies to combat infectious diseases.

Next, we provide an overview of NAbs for preventing infections in recent years. The initial success in targeting HIV was achieved with CD4-Fc fusion antibodies, which demonstrated highly effective anti-HIV responses. Given the absence of an HIV vaccine, the extraction of NAbs is crucial for treatment [95-97]. The primary target for NAbs against HIV is the viral glycoprotein envelope (ENV). Various NAbs have been developed based on the CD4 binding site of ENV [98-99], with some showing cross-neutralization against simian-human immunodeficiency virus (SHIV) [100-101]. To extend the half-life of NAbs, researchers have explored various delivery strategies with promising results. For examples in rhesus monkeys, AAV delivery of the NAbs-B12 genome achieved anti-HIV effects lasting up to six months [17]. Similarly, a single intramuscular injection of AAV1 encoding an antibody-like immunoadhesin molecule leads to the sustained expression of bioactive proteins that block SIV attack for over a year [102]. The following study linked the heavy and light chains of NAbs to viral peptide sequences. Subsequently, gene editing increased the AAV-mediated expression of NAbs to several-fold *in vivo* [17]. The B cell delivery system has also shown promise in the anti-HIV field. By genetically modifying B cells to highly express the HIV antibody 3BNC60, researchers observed a significant reduction in serum HIV levels in mice that demonstrated this delivery system's highly efficient neutralizing ability [66]. Recent advancements, such as identifying the *Fc* structural domain of HIV, have led to developing more potent HIV NAbs, including PG9, PG16, and VRC01, which exhibit tenfold greater potency than earlier antibodies [103-107]. The global COVID-19 pandemic has led to a high incidence of morbidity and mortality. The SARS-CoV-2-S is a significant target for NAbs. Designing NAbs specifically targeting the S protein's receptor-binding domain (RBD) has shown significant efficacy against SARS-CoV-2 [108]. Additionally, neutralizing mAbs targeting pro-inflammatory cytokines (IL-17, IL-6) may have a notable impact on SARS-CoV-2 [109]. The subsequent clinical trials demonstrated their effectiveness in controlling COVID-19 symptoms [110]. It has been demonstrated that CR3022 is the RBD-specific human neutralizing mAb initially developed for SARS-CoV-2 and exhibits high affinity for the SARS-CoV-2-RBD [39, 111]. Recent studies have further identified the S protein's N-terminal structural domain (NTD) as a promising target for therapeutic mAbs against COVID-19 [112]. Furthermore, NAbs against Middle East respiratory syndrome coronavirus and severe acute respiratory syndrome have shown favorable therapeutic outcomes. Transgenic mice treated with AAV vectors combined with three monoclonal antibodies (AR4A, AR3A, and AR3B) demonstrated complete resistance to HCV infection [71]. However, it is essential to consider that the affinity of SARS-CoV-2-NAbs receptors is relatively poor, and only a tiny fraction (0.1%) of NAbs can reach the respiratory mucosa after intravenous injection, limiting their therapeutic efficacy. Therefore, mucosal immune NAbs have garnered attention as a potential solution. Notably, NAbs treated by a vibrating mesh nebulizer retained their neutralizing activity effectively, and subsequent lung inhalation of IN-006 resulted in lung antibody levels up to 100 times higher than in serum. Furthermore, nasal inhalation of lgY and exosomes delivering RBD-mRNA have been explored as a potential treatment for COVID-19 [15, 113-114]. NAbs in the context of bacterial infections have received comparatively less attention, with the focus primarily directed towards the botulinum toxin infections and protective antigenic structural domain of Bacillus anthracis or Clostridioides difficile toxins [31, 115]. Botulinum toxin infections are caused by a potent neurotoxin produced by the bacterium Clostridium botulinum, which can lead to severe central and peripheral nervous system disorders. The botulinum neurotoxin (BoNT) has a high affinity for receptors on the presynaptic cell membrane at the neuromuscular junction. It exerts its effects by cleaving synaptic proteins and disrupting the release of acetylcholine neurotransmitter vesicles into the synaptic gap. As a result, the neuromuscular transmission fails and leads to various symptoms, such as muscle fatigue, eyelid ptosis, respiratory muscle paralysis and dysphagia. To counteract the detrimental effects of BoNT, botulinum toxin NAbs can be administered intravenously to bind to BoNT and block or inhibit its action at the presynaptic membrane or nerve terminals, which helps mitigate the impact of the neurotoxin [116-117]. Efforts have been made to explore antibodies that target the conserved haemagglutinin A stem region of Haemophilus influenzae. However, the development of effective antibodies in this regard has yet to be achieved.

Application of NAbs to Treat Cancers

NAbs have been extensively utilized in antitumor therapy, particularly in treating solid tumors and hematological diseases. Their application in oncology primarily involves inhibiting tumor growth and metastasis by inhibiting the binding of cell surface receptors. One of the critical therapeutic targets for antitumor monoclonal antibodies is the overexpression of growth factor receptors, such as epidermal growth factor receptors (EGFR) including EGFR and HER2. By neutralizing these receptors, the signaling pathways are disrupted and lead to reduced tumor growth and the induction of apoptosis [31, 118]. For examples, trastuzumab is an NAb that can effectively block HER2 signaling and is commonly used to treat HER2-positive breast cancer where HER2 is highly expressed [118]. Bevacizumab can target the vascular endothelial growth factor VEGF to inhibit tumor growth, but its systemic administration will cause hypertension, kidney failure and other side effects. Therefore, we choose inhalation as a non-invasive way of drug delivery. It can also be applied to various types of cancer while reducing the toxicity and side effects of bevacizumab [72].

NAbs can also act as immune effectors to mediate *Fc*-mediated immune responses against cells expressing specific targets. In addition to growth factor receptors, NAbs can also target glycoproteins such as CD20, CD30, CD33, and CD52, present on the surface of tumor cells. For example, rituximab binds to CD20, a B cell surface marker. Its *Fc* region interacts with *FcγR* expressed by immune cells, which could trigger inflammation, directly kill B cells, or lead to phagocytosis within the body [119-120]. However, it is crucial not to overlook the issue of the relatively short biological half-life of NAbs *in vivo*, which is attributed to immune clearance. To address this limitation and enhance the therapeutic efficacy of NAbs in cancer treatment, researchers have been exploring the use of delivery vectors and optimizing the route of administration. For example, one promising approach involves utilizing AAV as a delivery vehicle to transfer the HIL-15 gene, successfully expressing HIL-25 NAbs with potent anticancer effects. This strategy overcomes the need for frequent repeated administrations, offering a more sustainable and efficient treatment option [38]. Similarly, lipid nanoparticles have been employed to encapsulate NAbs-mRNA allowing for prolonged antiviral effects against the SARS-CoV-2 virus for up to 60 days [14]. These innovative delivery methods provide a prolonged and sustained release of NAbs, further improving their therapeutic potential. Moreover, NAbs can serve as immune checkpoint inhibitors by targeting immune cells. They primarily block cytotoxic T-lymphocyte-associated antigen 4 (CTLA-4) and programmed cell death protein 1 (PD-1). Ipilimumab (Yervoy) is a NAb against CTLA-4, and it has been approved for treating advanced melanoma. Nivolumab is an antibody targeting PD-1 and has demonstrated efficacy in various cancer types [31, 121-123].

Application of NAbs to Treat Inflammatory and Other Diseases

In addition to infectious diseases and cancer, NAbs are widely used in inflammatory arthritis, autoimmune diseases, and ocular diseases. In particular, the delivery pathway of NAbs plays an essential role in immunodeficiency diseases and ocular-targeted drug delivery.

Rheumatoid Arthritis (RA) is an autoimmune inflammatory disease affecting approximately 1% of adults and primarily affects the synovial membranes of multiple joints leading to symmetric synovitis. It is commonly observed in the metacarpophalangeal and proximal interphalangeal joints of the hands and feet [124]. The primary cell regulators targeting TNF-α and IL-6 have been extensively studied in treating RA. For example, Etanercept is an NAb of the human TNF-α receptor p75, produced through recombinant DNA technology using a Chinese hamster ovary (CHO) mammalian expression system. Clinical trials have demonstrated its efficacy in improving the condition of RA patients [125]. Tocilizumab and sarilumab are two mAbs against IL-6. Tocilizumab binds to IL-6 receptors, inhibits these receptor-mediated signaling, and is effective in rheumatoid arthritis in a short time [10]. In addition, TNF-a NAbs are used to treat inflammatory bowel disease. As the first reported TNF-α NAb for treating inflammatory bowel disease, infliximab received approval in 2002 for inducing and maintaining clinical remission in Crohn's disease [126-127]. Ustekinumab is a fully human IgG1 mAb that targets the shared p40 subunit of cytokines IL-12 and IL-23 and it has been demonstrated effective in treating Crohn's disease, psoriasis, and psoriatic arthritis [128]. Despite limited research on NAbs delivery in inflammatory arthritis diseases, the challenges of NAb instability and low bioavailability are noteworthy. Therefore, selecting appropriate delivery vehicles and administration routes holds significant promise for addressing these issues effectively. Berger et al. first reported using slow subcutaneous injection of 16.5% intramuscular immunoglobulin to replace antibodies in immunodeficient patients. Compared to intravenous injection, subcutaneous delivery was more manageable, better tolerated and reduced antibody toxicity. Similarly, Wakim et al. demonstrated that subcutaneous NAbs injection in immunodeficient patients achieved a drug exposure (area under the curve) comparable to intravenous administration. As subcutaneous injection requires lymphocyte-mediated entry into the circulatory system, peak NAb concentration was reached after four days resulting in reduced allergic reactions among patients. Therefore, subcutaneous injection provides extended drug circulation time and minimizes toxic side effects [129]. NAbs have also been approved for topical targeted delivery and other treatment approaches across various tissues. For example, ranibizumab is a topically active antibody fragment and has been approved for treating age-related wet macular degeneration. Intraocular targeted delivery of NAbs can overcome the ocular surface barrier by lens injection [130-131].

Conclusion

Due to numerous advantageous features (i.e., potent neutralizing activity and specificity) and potential for prophylactic and therapeutic applications, NAbs are gaining increasing prominence in scenarios where vaccines may not be feasible. However, several challenges still limit their full potential, such as short half-life, tissue specificity, immune response and dosing frequency. To overcome these limitations and enhance their therapeutic efficacy, researchers have explored a variety of delivery strategies and developed various routes of administration. AAV and lipid nanoparticles have shown promise in delivering the NAbs gene and prolonging circulation stability after a single dose. Exosomes and immune cells could protect NAbs from immune clearance, extending their biological half-life. Nasal-oral inhalation, intrathecal and len administration offer tissue and organ targeting capacity. Meanwhile, intramuscular and subcutaneous injections have gained popularity in terms of safety, convenience, and ease of administration. Tailoring the delivery vehicles and administration routes to meet specific therapeutic needs may significantly enhance the therapeutic efficacy of NAbs. Given that the transformation of NAbs critically depends on developing effective delivery strategies, further research on the delivery process and the underlying mechanisms is necessary. Additionally, it is essential to conduct in-depth studies to explore the immunoregulatory mechanism of delivery platforms to minimize immunogenicity. Moreover, considering the diversity of immune status and pathological characteristics among patients, personalized therapeutic strategies may help to unleash the full therapeutic potential of NAbs. Hence, further in-depth works on the delivery strategies and therapeutic application of NAbs are essential to advance the development of the field and optimize the effectiveness of NAbs for the prevention or treatment of different infections and diseases.

Acknowledgments

The authors thank the National Natural Science Foundation of China (32371440, 32101157, 82104105), National Key Research & Development Program of China (2023YFC2605000), and China Postdoctoral Science Foundation (2021M693966). M. L. and Q. L. conceived the content. M. L. led the project. Q. L. wrote the manuscript. H. X. and M. L. revised the manuscript. A. Z. and Y. H. gave important advices.

References

[1] Murin CD, Wilson IA, Ward AB. Antibody responses to viral infections: A structural perspective across three different enveloped viruses [J]. *Nat Microbiol,* 2019, 4: 734-747.

[2] Chen C, Liang J, Hu H, et al. Research progress in methods for detecting neutralizing antibodies against sars-cov-2 [J]. *Anal Biochem*, 2023, 673: 115199.

[3] Parkin J, Cohen B. An overview of the immune system [J]. *Lancet*, 2001, 357: 1777-1789.

[4] Ali MG, Zhang Z, Gao Q, et al. Recent advances in therapeutic applications of neutralizing antibodies for virus infections: An overview [J]. *Immunol Res*, 2020, 68: 325-339.

[5] Burton DR. Antiviral neutralizing antibodies: From in vitro to in vivo activity [J]. *Nat Rev Immunol*, 2023, 17: 1-15.

[6] Koff WC, Burton DR, Johnson PR, et al. Accelerating next-generation vaccine development for global disease prevention [J]. *Science*, 2013, 340: 1232910.

[7] Krause PR, Bialek SR, Boppana SB, et al. Priorities for cmv vaccine development [J]. *Vaccine*, 2013, 32: 4-10.

[8] Garrone P, Fluckiger AC, Mangeot PE, et al. A prime-boost strategy using virus-like particles pseudotyped for hcv proteins triggers broadly neutralizing antibodies in macaques [J]. *Sci Transl Med*, 2011, 3:71-94.

[9] Mascola JR, Montefiori DC. The role of antibodies in hiv vaccines [J]. *Annu Rev Immunol*, 2010, 28: 413-444.

[10] Posner J, Barrington P, Brier T, et al. Monoclonal antibodies: Past, present and future [J]. *Handb Exp Pharmacol*, 2019, 260: 81-141.

[11] Yang X, Bian J, Wang Z, et al. A bio-liposome activating natural killer cell by illuminating tumor homogenization antigen properties [J]. *Adv Sci* (Weinh), 2023, 10: e2205449.

[12] Carnasciali A, Amoriello R, Bonechi E, et al. T cell delivery of nanoparticles-bound anti-cd20 monoclonal antibody: Successful b cell depletion in the spinal cord during experimental autoimmune encephalomyelitis [J]. *J Neuroimmune Pharmacol*, 2021, 16: 376-389.

[13] Martinez-Navio JM, Fuchs SP, Pedreño-López S, et al. Host anti-antibody responses following adeno-associated virus-mediated delivery of antibodies against HIV and SIV in rhesus monkeys [J]. *Mol Ther*, 2016, 24: 76-86.

[14] Deng YQ, Zhang NN, Zhang YF, et al. Lipid nanoparticle-encapsulated mrna antibody provides long-term protection against sars-cov-2 in mice and hamsters [J]. *Cell Res,* 2022, 32: 375-382.

[15] Zhang Q, Wang M, Han C, et al. Intraduodenal delivery of exosome-loaded sars-cov-2 rbd mrna induces a neutralizing antibody response in mice [J]. *Vaccines* (Basel), 2023, 11: 673.

[16] Aqil F, Munagala R, Jeyabalan J, et al. Milk exosomes - natural nanoparticles for sirna delivery [J]. *Cancer Lett*, 2019, 449: 186-195.

[17] Joshi LR, Gálvez NMS, Ghosh S, et al. Delivery platforms for broadly neutralizing antibodies [J]. *Curr Opin HIV AIDS*, 2023, 18: 191-208.

[18] McCarty DM, Monahan PE, Samulski RJ. Self-complementary recombinant adeno-associated virus (scaav) vectors promote efficient transduction independently of DNA synthesis [J]. *Gene Ther*, 2001, 8: 1248-1254.

[19] Schnepp BC, Johnson PR. Adeno-associated virus delivery of broadly neutralizing antibodies [J]. *Curr Opin HIV AIDS*, 2014, 9: 250-256.

[20] Piepenbrink MS, Park JG, Oladunni FS, et al. Therapeutic activity of an inhaled potent sars-cov-2 neutralizing human monoclonal antibody in hamsters [J]. *Cell Rep Med*, 2021, 2: 100218.

[21] Micheli L, Parisio C, Lucarini E, et al. Vegf-a/vegfr-1 signalling and chemotherapy-induced neuropathic pain: Therapeutic potential of a novel anti-vegfr-1 monoclonal antibody [J]. *J Exp Clin Cancer Res*, 2021, 40: 320.

[22] Bodier-Montagutelli E, Respaud R, Watier H, et al. Mabdelivery: Administration routes for antibody therapy third labex mabimprove industrial workshop, july 2, 2015 tours, france [J]. *MAbs,* 2017, 9: 579-585.

[23] Abela IA, Kadelka C, Trkola A. Correlates of broadly neutralizing antibody development [J]. *Curr Opin HIV AIDS*, 2019, 14: 279-285.

[24] Plotkin SA. Correlates of protection induced by vaccination [J]. *Clin Vaccine Immunol*, 2010, 17: 1055-1065.

[25] Suzuki M, Kato C, Kato A. Therapeutic antibodies: Their mechanisms of action and the pathological findings they induce in toxicity studies [J]. *J Toxicol Pathol*, 2015, 28: 133-139.

[26] Coënon L, Villalba M. From cd16a biology to antibody-dependent cell-mediated cytotoxicity improvement [J]. *Front Immunol*, 2022, 13: 913215.

[27] Pinto S, Pahl J, Schottelius A, et al. Reimagining antibody-dependent cellular cytotoxicity in cancer: The potential of natural killer cell engagers [J]. *Trends Immunol*, 2022, 43: 932-946.

[28] Zafir-Lavie I, Michaeli Y, Reiter Y. Novel antibodies as anticancer agents [J]. *Oncogene*, 2007, 26: 3714-3733.

[29] Kostova V, Désos P, Starck JB, et al. The chemistry behind adcs [J]. *Pharmaceuticals* (Basel), 2021, 14: 442.

[30] Leyva-Grado VH, Tan GS, Leon PE, et al. Direct administration in the respiratory tract improves efficacy of broadly neutralizing anti-influenza virus monoclonal antibodies [J]. *Antimicrob Agents Chemother*, 2015, 59: 4162-4172.

[31] Castelli MS, McGonigle P, Hornby PJ. The pharmacology and therapeutic applications of monoclonal antibodies [J]. *Pharmacol Res Perspect*, 2019, 7: e00535.

[32] Beccari MV, Mogle BT, Sidman EF, et al. Ibalizumab, a novel monoclonal antibody for the management of multidrug-resistant hiv-1 infection [J]. *Antimicrob Agents Chemother*, 2019, 63: e00110-19.

[33] Song R, Franco D, Kao CY, et al. Epitope mapping of ibalizumab, a humanized anti-cd4 monoclonal antibody with anti-hiv-1 activity in infected patients [J]. *J Virol,* 2010, 84: 6935-6942.

[34] Hurt AC, Wheatley AK. Neutralizing antibody therapeutics for covid-19 [J]. *Viruses*, 2021, 13.

[35] Chen P, Nirula A, Heller B, et al. Sars-cov-2 neutralizing antibody ly-cov555 in outpatients with covid-19 [J]. *N Engl J Med*, 2021, 384: 229-237.

[36] Cao Y, Jian F, Zhang Z, et al. Rational identification of potent and broad sarbecovirus-neutralizing antibody cocktails from sars convalescents [J]. *Cell Rep,* 2022, 41: 111845.

[37] Glassy MC, McKnight ME. Requirements for human antibody cocktails for oncology [J]. *Expert Opin Biol Ther*, 2005, 5: 1333-1338.

[38] Yiang GT, Chou PL, Tsai HF, et al. Immunotherapy for sv40 t/t antigen-induced breast cancer by recombinant adeno-associated virus serotype 2 carrying interleukin-15 in mice [J]. *Int J Mol Med*, 2012, 29: 809-814.

[39] Tian X, Li C, Huang A, et al. Potent binding of 2019 novel coronavirus spike protein by a sars coronavirus-specific human monoclonal antibody [J]. *Emerg Microbes Infect*, 2020, 9: 382-385.

[40] Wang N, Eerdun G, Dong Y, et al. Correlation of serum resistin level and other metabolic hormones and immune function in neonatal umbilical cord blood [J]. *Medicine* (Baltimore), 2021, 100: e25195.

[41] Shinkura R. Gut iga puts pathogens under pressure [J]. *Nat Microbiol*, 2021, 6: 826-827.

[42] Napodano C, Marino M, Stefanile A, et al. Immunological role of igg subclasses [J]. *Immunol Invest*, 2021, 50: 427-444.

[43] Pang X, Huang Z, Zhong T, et al. Cadonilimab, a tetravalent pd-1/ctla-4 bispecific antibody with trans-binding and enhanced target binding avidity [J]. *MAbs*, 2023, 15: 2180794.

[44] Gilbert PB, Huang Y, deCamp AC, et al. Neutralization titer biomarker for antibody-mediated prevention of hiv-1 acquisition [J]. *Nat Med*, 2022, 28: 1924-1932.

[45] Berns KI, Linden RM. The cryptic life style of adeno-associated virus [J]. *Bioessays*, 1995, 17: 237-245.

[46] Ellis BL, Hirsch ML, Barker JC, et al. A survey of ex vivo/in vitro transduction efficiency of mammalian primary cells and cell lines with nine natural adeno-

associated virus (aav1-9) and one engineered adeno-associated virus serotype [J]. *Virol J*, 2013, 10: 1743-422X.

[47] Bartel MA, Weinstein JR, Schaffer DV. Directed evolution of novel adeno-associated viruses for therapeutic gene delivery [J]. *Gene Ther*, 2012, 19: 694-700.

[48] Akbarzadeh A, Rezaei-Sadabady R, Davaran S, et al. Liposome: Classification, preparation, and applications [J]. *Nanoscale Res Lett*, 2013, 8: 102.

[49] Baumgart T, Hess ST, Webb WW. Imaging coexisting fluid domains in biomembrane models coupling curvature and line tension [J]. *Nature*, 2003, 425: 821-824.

[50] Keller CA, Kasemo B. Surface specific kinetics of lipid vesicle adsorption measured with a quartz crystal microbalance [J]. *Biophys J*, 1998, 75: 1397-1402.

[51] Kose N, Fox JM, Sapparapu G, et al. A lipid-encapsulated mrna encoding a potently neutralizing human monoclonal antibody protects against chikungunya infection [J]. *Sci Immu*nol, 2019,17: eaaw6647.

[52] Pardi N, Secreto AJ, Shan X, et al. Administration of nucleoside-modified mrna encoding broadly neutralizing antibody protects humanized mice from hiv-1 challenge [J]. *Nat Commun*, 2017, 8: 14630.

[53] Erasmus JH, Archer J, Fuerte-Stone J, et al. Intramuscular delivery of replicon rna encoding zikv-117 human monoclonal antibody protects against zika virus infection [J]. *Mol Ther Methods Clin Dev*, 2020, 18: 402-414.

[54] Gilchuk P, Bombardi RG, Erasmus JH, et al. Integrated pipeline for the accelerated discovery of antiviral antibody therapeutics [J]. *Nat Biomed Eng*, 2020, 4: 1030-1043.

[55] Van Hoecke L, Verbeke R, De Vlieger D, et al. Mrna encoding a bispecific single domain antibody construct protects against influenza a virus infection in mice [J]. *Mol Ther Nucleic Acids*, 2020, 20: 777-787.

[56] Lu M, Xing H, Xun Z, et al. Exosome-based small rna delivery: Progress and prospects [J]. *Asian J Pharm Sci*, 2018, 13: 1-11.

[57] Zhang W, Huang Q, Xiao W, et al. Advances in anti-tumor treatments targeting the cd47/sirpα axis [J]. *Front Immunol*, 2020, 11: 18.

[58] Yuan D, Zhao Y, Banks WA, et al. Macrophage exosomes as natural nanocarriers for protein delivery to inflamed brain [J]. *Biomaterials*, 2017, 142: 1-12.

[59] van den Boorn JG, Schlee M, Coch C, et al. Sirna delivery with exosome nanoparticles [J]. *Nat Biotechnol*, 2011, 29: 325-326.

[60] Kuate S, Cinatl J, Doerr HW, et al. Exosomal vaccines containing the s protein of the sars coronavirus induce high levels of neutralizing antibodies [J]. *Virology*, 2007, 362: 26-37.

[61] Wang Z, Popowski KD, Zhu D, et al. Exosomes decorated with a recombinant sars-cov-2 receptor-binding domain as an inhalable covid-19 vaccine [J]. *Nat Biomed Eng*, 2022, 6: 791-805.

[62] Jiang L, Driedonks TAP, Jong WSP, et al. A bacterial extracellular vesicle-based intranasal vaccine against sars-cov-2 protects against disease and elicits neutralizing antibodies to wild-type and delta variants [J]. *J Extracell Vesicles,* 2022, 11: e12192.

[63] Luo XM, Maarschalk E, O'Connell RM, et al. Engineering human hematopoietic stem/progenitor cells to produce a broadly neutralizing anti-hiv antibody after in vitro maturation to human b lymphocytes [J]. *Blood*, 2009, 113: 1422-1431.
[64] Fusil F, Calattini S, Amirache F, et al. A lentiviral vector allowing physiologically regulated membrane-anchored and secreted antibody expression depending on b-cell maturation status [J]. *Mol Ther*, 2015, 23: 1734-1747.
[65] Hung KL, Meitlis I, Hale M, et al. Engineering protein-secreting plasma cells by homology-directed repair in primary human b cells [J]. *Mol Ther*, 2018, 26: 456-467.
[66] Hartweger H, McGuire AT, Horning M, et al. Hiv-specific humoral immune responses by crispr/cas9-edited b cells [J]. *J Exp Med*, 2019, 216: 1301-1310.
[67] Vamva E, Ozog S, Leaman DP, et al. A lentiviral vector b cell gene therapy platform for the delivery of the anti-hiv-1 ecd4-ig-knob-in-hole-reversed immunoadhesin [J]. *Mol Ther Methods Clin Dev*, 2023, 28: 366-384.
[68] Chigutsa E, O'Brien L, Ferguson-Sells L, et al. Population pharmacokinetics and pharmacodynamics of the neutralizing antibodies bamlanivimab and etesevimab in patients with mild to moderate covid-19 infection [J]. *Clin Pharmacol Ther*, 2021, 110: 1302-1310.
[69] Julg B, Stephenson KE, Wagh K, et al. Safety and antiviral activity of triple combination broadly neutralizing monoclonal antibody therapy against hiv-1: A phase 1 clinical trial [J]. *Nat Med*, 2022, 28: 1288-1296.
[70] Mühe J, Aye PP, Quink C, et al. Neutralizing antibodies against epstein-barr virus infection of b cells can protect from oral viral challenge in the rhesus macaque animal model [J]. *Cell Rep Med*, 2021, 2: 100352.
[71] Julg B, Sok D, Schmidt SD, et al. Protective efficacy of broadly neutralizing antibodies with incomplete neutralization activity against simian-human immunodeficiency virus in rhesus monkeys [J]. *J Virol*, 2017, 91: e01187-17.
[72] Parray HA, Shukla S, Perween R, et al. Inhalation monoclonal antibody therapy: A new way to treat and manage respiratory infections [J]. *Appl Microbiol Biotechnol*, 2021, 105: 6315-6332.
[73] Levin MJ, Ustianowski A, De Wit S, et al. Intramuscular azd7442 (tixagevimab-cilgavimab) for prevention of covid-19 [J]. *N Engl J Med*, 2022, 386: 2188-2200.
[74] Del Rosario JMM, Smith M, Zaki K, et al. Protection from influenza by intramuscular gene vector delivery of a broadly neutralizing nanobody does not depend on antibody dependent cellular cytotoxicity [J]. *Front Immunol*, 2020, 11: 627.
[75] Keller MA, Stiehm ER. Passive immunity in prevention and treatment of infectious diseases [J]. *Clin Microbiol Rev*, 2000, 13: 602-614.
[76] Stiehm ER, Keller MA, Vyas GN. Preparation and use of therapeutic antibodies primarily of human origin [J]. *Biologicals*, 2008, 36: 363-374.
[77] Cruz-Teran C, Tiruthani K, McSweeney M, et al. Challenges and opportunities for antiviral monoclonal antibodies as covid-19 therapy [J]. *Adv Drug Deliv Rev*, 2021, 169: 100-117.

[78] Halwe S, Kupke A, Vanshylla K, et al. Intranasal administration of a monoclonal neutralizing antibody protects mice against sars-cov-2 infection [J]. *Viruses*, 2021, 13: 1498.

[79] Ku Z, Xie X, Hinton PR, et al. Nasal delivery of an igm offers broad protection from sars-cov-2 variants [J]. *Nature*, 2021, 595: 718-723.

[80] Prince GA, Hemming VG, Horswood RL, et al. Effectiveness of topically administered neutralizing antibodies in experimental immunotherapy of respiratory syncytial virus infection in cotton rats [J]. *J Virol*, 1987, 61: 1851-1854.

[81] Weltzin R, Traina-Dorge V, Soike K, et al. Intranasal monoclonal iga antibody to respiratory syncytial virus protects rhesus monkeys against upper and lower respiratory tract infection [J]. *J Infect Dis*, 1996, 174: 256-261.

[82] Ladel S, Flamm J, Zadeh AS, et al. Allogenic fc domain-facilitated uptake of igg in nasal lamina propria: Friend or foe for intranasal cns delivery? [J]. *Pharmaceutics*, 2018, 10: 107.

[83] Ladel S, Maigler F, Flamm J, et al. Impact of glycosylation and species origin on the uptake and permeation of iggs through the nasal airway mucosa [J]. *Pharmaceutics*, 2020, 12: 1014.

[84] Yoshida M, Claypool SM, Wagner JS, et al. Human neonatal fc receptor mediates transport of igg into luminal secretions for delivery of antigens to mucosal dendritic cells [J]. *Immunity*, 2004, 20: 769-783.

[85] Fatima N, Kaushik V, Ayoub A. A narrative review of a pulmonary aerosolized formulation or a nasal drop using sera containing neutralizing antibodies collected from covid-19-recovered patients as a probable therapy for covid-19 [J]. *Iran J Med Sci*, 2021, 46: 151-168.

[86] Li C, Zhan W, Yang Z, et al. Broad neutralization of sars-cov-2 variants by an inhalable bispecific single-domain antibody [J]. *Cell*, 2022, 185: 1389-1401.

[87] Li Q, Wang C, Hu J, et al. Cannabidiol-loaded biomimetic macrophage membrane vesicles against post-traumatic stress disorder assisted by ultrasound [J]. *Int J Pharm*, 2023, 637: 122872.

[88] Ericson T, Singla P, Kohan L. Intrathecal pumps [J]. *Phys Med Rehabil Clin N Am*, 2022, 33: 409-424.

[89] Brastianos PK, Lee EQ, Cohen JV, et al. Single-arm, open-label phase 2 trial of pembrolizumab in patients with leptomeningeal carcinomatosis [J]. *Nat Med*, 2020, 26: 1280-1284.

[90] Koike K, Beatman EL, Schweitzer KS, et al. Subcutaneous administration of neutralizing antibodies to endothelial monocyte-activating protein ii attenuates cigarette smoke-induced lung injury in mice [J]. *Am J Physiol Lung Cell Mol Physiol*, 2019, 316: L558-l566.

[91] Berger M. Subcutaneous immunoglobulin replacement in primary immunodeficiencies [J]. *Clin Immunol*, 2004, 112: 1-7.

[92] Berger M, Cupps TR, Fauci AS. Immunoglobulin replacement therapy by slow subcutaneous infusion [J]. *Ann Intern Med*, 1980, 93: 55-56.

[93] Caskey M, Klein F, Lorenzi JC, et al. Viraemia suppressed in hiv-1-infected humans by broadly neutralizing antibody 3bnc117 [J]. *Nature*, 2015, 522: 487-491.

[94] Wang J, Shao Y, Wang W, et al. Caspase-11 deficiency impairs neutrophil recruitment and bacterial clearance in the early stage of pulmonary klebsiella pneumoniae infection [J]. *Int J Med Microbiol*, 2017, 307: 490-496.

[95] Czajkowsky DM, Hu J, Shao Z, et al. Fc-fusion proteins: New developments and future perspectives [J]. *EMBO Mol Med*, 2012, 4: 1015-1028.

[96] Gautam R, Nishimura Y, Gaughan N, et al. A single injection of crystallizable fragment domain-modified antibodies elicits durable protection from shiv infection [J]. *Nat Med*, 2018, 24: 610-616.

[97] Walker LM, Huber M, Doores KJ, et al. Broad neutralization coverage of hiv by multiple highly potent antibodies [J]. *Nature*, 2011, 477: 466-470.

[98] Freund NT, Wang H, Scharf L, et al. Coexistence of potent hiv-1 broadly neutralizing antibodies and antibody-sensitive viruses in a viremic controller [J]. *Sci Transl Med*, 2017, 9: eaal2144.

[99] Liao HX, Lynch R, Zhou T, et al. Co-evolution of a broadly neutralizing hiv-1 antibody and founder virus [J]. *Nature*, 2013, 496: 469-476.

[100] Han Q, Jones JA, Nicely NI, et al. Difficult-to-neutralize global hiv-1 isolates are neutralized by antibodies targeting open envelope conformations [J]. *Nat Commun*, 2019, 10: 2898.

[101] Shingai M, Donau OK, Plishka RJ, et al. Passive transfer of modest titers of potent and broadly neutralizing anti-hiv monoclonal antibodies block shiv infection in macaques [J]. *J Exp Med*, 2014, 211: 2061-2074.

[102] Johnson PR, Schnepp BC, Zhang J, et al. Vector-mediated gene transfer engenders long-lived neutralizing activity and protection against siv infection in monkeys [J]. *Nat Med*, 2009, 15: 901-906.

[103] Molinos-Albert LM, Clotet B, Blanco J, et al. Immunologic insights on the membrane proximal external region: A major human immunodeficiency virus type-1 vaccine target [J]. *Front Immunol*, 2017, 8: 1154.

[104] DiLillo DJ, Tan GS, Palese P, et al. Broadly neutralizing hemagglutinin stalk-specific antibodies require fcγr interactions for protection against influenza virus in vivo [J]. *Nat Med*, 2014, 20: 143-151.

[105] Walker LM, Phogat SK, Chan-Hui PY, et al. Broad and potent neutralizing antibodies from an african donor reveal a new hiv-1 vaccine target [J]. *Science*, 2009, 326: 285-289.

[106] Wu X, Yang ZY, Li Y, et al. Rational design of envelope identifies broadly neutralizing human monoclonal antibodies to hiv-1 [J]. *Science*, 2010, 329: 856-861.

[107] Hartman AL, Towner JS, Nichol ST. Ebola and marburg hemorrhagic fever [J]. *Clin Lab Med*, 2010, 30: 161-177.

[108] Shanmugaraj B, Siriwattananon K, Wangkanont K, et al. Perspectives on monoclonal antibody therapy as potential therapeutic intervention for coronavirus disease-19 (covid-19) [J]. *Asian Pac J Allergy Immunol*, 2020, 38: 10-18.

[109] Tan M, Liu Y, Zhou R, et al. Immunopathological characteristics of coronavirus disease 2019 cases in guangzhou, china [J]. *Immunology*, 2020, 160: 261-268.

[110] Cao X. Covid-19: Immunopathology and its implications for therapy [J]. *Nat Rev Immunol*, 2020, 20: 269-270.

[111] Rogers TF, Zhao F, Huang D, et al. Isolation of potent sars-cov-2 neutralizing antibodies and protection from disease in a small animal model [J]. *Science*, 2020, 369: 956-963.

[112] Chi X, Yan R, Zhang J, et al. A neutralizing human antibody binds to the n-terminal domain of the spike protein of sars-cov-2 [J]. *Science*, 2020, 369: 650-655.

[113] McSweeney MD, Stewart I, Richardson Z, et al. Stable nebulization and muco-trapping properties of regdanvimab/in-006 support its development as a potent, dose-saving inhaled therapy for covid-19 [J]. *Bioeng Transl Med*, 2022, 8: e10391.

[114] Focosi D, McConnell S, Casadevall A, et al. Monoclonal antibody therapies against sars-cov-2 [J]. *Lancet Infect Dis*, 2022, 22: e311-e326.

[115] Henning LN, Carpenter S, Stark GV, et al. Development of protective immunity in new zealand white rabbits challenged with bacillus anthracis spores and treated with antibiotics and obiltoxaximab, a monoclonal antibody against protective antigen [J]. *Antimicrob Agents Chemother*, 2018, 62: e01590-17.

[116] Chalk CH, Benstead TJ, Pound JD, et al. Medical treatment for botulism [J]. *Cochrane Database Syst Rev*, 2019, 4: CD008123.

[117] Wendt S, Eder I, Wölfel R, et al. [botulism: Diagnosis and therapy] [J]. *Dtsch Med Wochenschr*, 2017, 142: 1304-1312.

[118] Weiner LM, Surana R, Wang S. Monoclonal antibodies: Versatile platforms for cancer immunotherapy [J]. *Nat Rev Immunol*, 2010, 10: 317-327.

[119] Davis TA, Czerwinski DK, Levy R. Therapy of b-cell lymphoma with anti-cd20 antibodies can result in the loss of cd20 antigen expression [J]. *Clin Cancer Res*, 1999, 5: 611-615.

[120] Lim SH, Beers SA, French RR, et al. Anti-cd20 monoclonal antibodies: Historical and future perspectives [J]. *Haematologica*, 2010, 95: 135-143.

[121] Kimiz-Gebologlu I, Gulce-Iz S, Biray-Avci C. Monoclonal antibodies in cancer immunotherapy [J]. *Mol Biol Rep*, 2018, 45: 2935-2940.

[122] Topalian SL, Taube JM, Anders RA, et al. Mechanism-driven biomarkers to guide immune checkpoint blockade in cancer therapy [J]. *Nat Rev Cancer*, 2016, 16: 275-287.

[123] Gong J, Chehrazi-Raffle A, Reddi S, et al. Development of pd-1 and pd-l1 inhibitors as a form of cancer immunotherapy: A comprehensive review of registration trials and future considerations [J]. *J Immunother Cancer*, 2018, 6: 8.

[124] Scott DL, Wolfe F, Huizinga TW. Rheumatoid arthritis [J]. *Lancet*, 2010, 376: 1094-1108.

[125] Bathon JM, Martin RW, Fleischmann RM, et al. A comparison of etanercept and methotrexate in patients with early rheumatoid arthritis [J]. *N Engl J Med*, 2000, 343: 1586-1593.

[126] Targan SR, Hanauer SB, van Deventer SJ, et al. A short-term study of chimeric monoclonal antibody ca2 to tumor necrosis factor alpha for crohn's disease. Crohn's disease ca2 study group [J]. *N Engl J Med*, 1997, 337: 1029-1035.

[127] Behm BW, Bickston SJ. Tumor necrosis factor-alpha antibody for maintenance of remission in crohn's disease [J]. *Cochrane Database Syst Rev*, 2008: CD006893.

[128] Feagan BG, Sandborn WJ, Gasink C, et al. Ustekinumab as induction and maintenance therapy for crohn's disease [J]. *N Engl J Med*, 2016, 375: 1946-1960.

[129] Stiehm ER, Casillas AM, Finkelstein JZ, et al. Slow subcutaneous human intravenous immunoglobulin in the treatment of antibody immunodeficiency: Use of an old method with a new product [J]. *J Allergy Clin Immunol*, 1998, 101: 848-849.

[130] Knödler M, Körfer J, Kunzmann V, et al. Randomised phase ii trial to investigate catumaxomab (anti-epcam × anti-cd3) for treatment of peritoneal carcinomatosis in patients with gastric cancer [J]. *Br J Cancer*, 2018, 119: 296-302.

[131] Bakri SJ, Snyder MR, Reid JM, et al. Pharmacokinetics of intravitreal ranibizumab (lucentis) [J]. *Ophthalmology*, 2007, 114: 2179-2182.

Chapter 3

Neutralizing Antibodies against Enterovirus: Recent Advances and Future Challenges

Longfa Xu[*,†]
Rui Zhu[*]
and Tong Cheng
State Key Laboratory of Molecular Vaccinology and Molecular Diagnostics,
National Institute of Diagnostics and Vaccine Development in Infectious Diseases,
School of Public Health, School of Life Sciences, Xiamen University, Xiamen, PR China
Xiang An Biomedicine Laboratory, Xiamen, China
Research Unit of Frontier Technology of Structural Vaccinology,
Chinese Academy of Medical Sciences, Xiamen Fujian, China

Abstract

Enteroviral infections continue to cause morbidity and mortality in susceptible individuals worldwide. However, effective antiviral drugs or vaccines remain lacking in targeting most circulating enteroviruses. Antibody-mediated immunity plays a crucial role in preventing and limiting enteroviral infections. This review primarily focuses on enteroviruses that have caused recent endemics, including poliovirus, enterovirus A71 (EV-A71), coxsackievirus and rhinovirus. Additionally, we provide an insightful analysis of the structural mechanisms underlying virus neutralization. The mechanisms underlying the neutralization of enteroviruses by type-specific antibodies have been demonstrated to target different steps of the viral infection cascade, including blocking virion-receptor interactions, inducing premature

[*] Authors equally contributed to this work.
[†] Corresponding Author's Email: longfaxu@xmu.edu.cn.

In: Neutralizing Antibodies and their Role in Health and Disease
Editors: Chenguang Shen, Yang Yang and Minghui Yang
ISBN: 979-8-89113-541-3

uncoating of virions via functional mimicry, or destabilizing the capsid and inducing virion disruption. These type-specific neutralizing antibodies have demonstrated the ability to target multiple antigenic loops, recognize distinct viral conformations, and offer protective effects solely against a limited subset of viruses. Moreover, this review also discusses recent advances in the relative importance of Fc-dependent effector functions and the structural rearrangements that occur during the antibody cocktail. These findings offer valuable insights into the potential mechanisms underlying enterovirus neutralization.

Keywords: enterovirus, virus uncoating, neutralizing antibody, epitope

Introduction

Human Enterovirus (HEV) belongs to the *Picornaviridae* family, a group of small RNA viruses, which includes 4 types of enteroviruses (A to D) and 3 types of rhinoviruses (A to C) [1]. In addition to the three poliovirus serotypes, these seven species encompass over 250 other types. These enteroviruses encompass several significant pathogens, including coxsackieviruses, echoviruses, numbered enteroviruses and rhinoviruses. They infect millions of people worldwide each year and have the potential to cause a diverse array of disorders with varying presentation and severity, particularly in infants, young children, and immunocompromised individuals. They typically manifest as either asymptomatic or mild and self-limiting symptoms after infection. These symptoms often include fever, respiratory symptoms (such as cough, wheezing and sore throat), gastrointestinal symptoms (vomiting, diarrhea), and/or hand, foot, and mouth disease (HFMD) [2, 3]. In a small number of cases, severe infections may occur, leading to aseptic meningitis, encephalitis, acute flaccid paralysis, acute flaccid myelitis, myocarditis and neonatal sepsis [4, 5]. The clinical presentation of severe infections is highly correlated with age, and approximately 58% of infants and children diagnosed with meningitis/encephalitis and 52% of infected adults with this condition are caused by enteroviruses, which are the most common etiology of meningitis/encephalitis [6, 7]. HFMD is one of the most common manifestations of enterovirus infections. Many pathogenic subtypes of enteroviruses causing this disease have neurotropic properties, such as Enterovirus A71 (EV-A71), Coxsackievirus A6 (CV-A6), CV-A10, CV-A16, CV-B1 CV-B3 and so on, which have been confirmed to be involved in central nervous system infections. Coxsackievirus B-group viruses, especially CV-

B3, are widely recognized to be associated with myocarditis [8]. CV-Bs and echoviruses are also implicated as environmental factors in the etiology of type 1 diabetes through persistent infection and inflammation of pancreatic β-cells [9]. Rhinoviruses cause the common cold, but they can also trigger severe respiratory tract diseases and exacerbate asthma and chronic obstructive pulmonary disease (COPD) [10, 11]. Enteroviruses, despite their name and the fact that they are transmitted through the fecal-oral route, are not associated with gastrointestinal illnesses. Aside from three marketed inactivated EVA71 vaccines in China [12-14], no effective preventive or therapeutic measures are available for enterovirus infections.

The enterovirus capsids comprise 60 copies of four viral proteins: VP1, VP2, VP3, and VP4 [1]. These proteins are arranged with pseudo $T = 3$ symmetry [15, 16]. VP1, VP2, and VP3 make up the outer surface of the capsid and have a β-sandwich jelly roll fold, while VP4 is situated in an extended conformation on the inner surface of the capsid. The icosahedral 5-fold axes of the capsid feature a deep surface depression called a "canyon," which contains the receptor-binding site [17]. Enteroviruses use a diverse range of receptors and endocytic routes [1]. However, the uncoating mechanism follows a series of conserved steps that gradually destabilize the virus particle and result in the release of its genome. Several primary forms of the enterovirus particle have been identified throughout its life cycle, including the procapsid, mature virion, A-particle and empty particle [1]. The structure of the mature virion is dynamic and undergoes a process known as "breathing," characterized by periodic expansions and contractions of the virion. During this process, VP4 and the N-terminal extension of VP1 are transiently exposed [18, 19]. Cellular cues, such as receptor binding or low endosomal pH, can trigger a sequence of conformational changes in the capsid, including the collapse of the pocket and conformational alterations at receptor-binding sites [20-22]. These changes ultimately lead to an expanded uncoating intermediate or A-particle.

There are no approved licensed vaccines or antiviral drugs against most circulating enteroviruses. Antibody-based immunity prevents and limits enteroviral infections [23, 24]. Specifically, virus neutralization is primarily achieved through the action of specific antibodies. Recent progress in elucidating viral structures and antibody-virus complexes has dramatically enhanced our understanding of this neutralization mechanism. Furthermore, identifying and characterizing potent monoclonal antibodies enables researchers to determine the relevant neutralization epitopes at the molecular level. In this review, we will focus on enteroviruses that have been circulating and causing outbreaks in endemic regions over the past decade while introducing the current molecular understanding of the structure-based neutralization mechanism of antibodies and also the relative importance of Fc-dependent effector functions and the structural rearrangements that occur during the antibody cocktail.

Neutralizing by Viral Capsid Stabilization

Antibody-mediated neutralization *in vitro* against human enteroviruses is increasingly understood to operate by various mechanisms. Antibodies that bind with sufficient affinity to a native structure on virions can potentially interfere with viral entry. Dozens of monoclonal antibodies (mAbs) have been found to neutralize viruses by capsid stabilization and /or blocking receptor binding (Table 1). These antibodies target either the known viral receptor binding domains directly or partially, or they bind to regions adjacent to the receptors, thereby impeding viral-receptor binding through steric obstruction. Enteroviruses can bind to a large repertoire of different receptors specifically categorized as attachment and uncoating receptors, and the binding regions on virions for various receptors show significant differences. For EV-A71 and CV-A16, three major distinct receptors have been identified: scavenger receptor class B member 2 (SCARB2) [25, 26], P-selectin glycoprotein ligand 1 (PSGL-1) [27, 28] and heparan sulfate (HS) [29, 30]. SCARB2 serves as the canyon-binding receptor with the dominating binding site of the VP1 GH and VP2 EF loops [31]. Neutralizing antibodies (nAbs), including 22A12 [32, 33], D5 [34], D6 [35], 38-1-10A [36] and 38-3-11A [36] against EV-A71, as well as NA9D7 [37], 14B10 [37] and 8C4 [38] against CV-A16, have been validated to efficiently block or interfere with the virus-SCARB2 interaction. The others (MA28-7 [39] and E1 [40] against EV-A71, 18A7 [37] and 9B5 [38] against CV-A16 could neutralize virus infection via inhibiting the interactions with PSGL-1 and/or HS, binding at the 5-fold vertex. Specifically, 14B10 and NA9D7 against CV-A16 exhibited potent neutralization activities and therapeutic potential, and bind exclusively to mature virions surrounding viral 3-fold and 2-fold vertices, respectively (Table 1). The two nAbs recognized protective epitopes that could overlap with the SCARB2-binding sites [37]. Additionally, KREMEN1 has been identified as an entry receptor for additional human type A enteroviruses (HEV-As), including CV-A10 [41, 42]. A potent antibody, named 2G8, was further obtained and exhibited strong preventive and therapeutic efficacy against CVA10 infection [43]. 2G8 binds at a border region spanning all three viral proteins (VP1 to VP3) at the quasi-3-fold vertex (Table 1), and cross-reacts with three forms of capsids. Overlaying 2G8 with CV-A10/KREMEN1 has shown severe clashes between the Fabs and receptor, with no antibody-induced conformational change within the capsid, suggesting that neutralization is mainly mediated by preventing receptor attachment.

For human type B enterovirus (HEV-B), coxsackievirus and adenovirus receptor (CAR) is the universal uncoating receptor of CV-B1 to CV-B6 [44]. Three CV-B1-specific neutralizing antibodies that targeted CAR-binding sites, named 2E6, 8A10 and 9A3, were generated and identified with the ability to inhibit receptor engagement [45]. High-resolution cryo-electron microscopy (cryo-EM) structures revealed that these antibodies bound to distinct epitopes but with an overlapping region in the capsid VP2 protein, particularly within the highly variable EF loop [45]. As with many other HEV-Bs, Echoviruses (E) are thought to utilize two types of receptors to infect cells: the decay-accelerating factor (DAF/CD55) for viral attachment [46], and the neonatal Fc receptor (FcRn) for viral uncoating [47, 48]. Several highly potent antibodies, including 6C5 [49] and 4B10 [49] against E30, as well as 5G3 [50] and 6D10 [51] against E3, could efficiently block viral binding to their receptors. 6C5 and 4B10 engage the capsid loci at the canyon's and in-canyon's north rim, respectively. At the same time, 5G3 and 6D10 target similar epitopes surrounding the 2-fold vertex that are close to but have no significant overlap with the receptor-binding sites (Table 1). Thus, the ability of 5G3/6D10 to prevent E3 from binding with receptors can be attributed to the steric clashes caused by proximal overlapping binding sites. Furthermore, the chimpanzee anti-poliovirus antibody A12 [52] and four VHHs (PVSP29F, PVSP19B, PVSP6A and PVSS8A) [53] could also neutralize viruses by capsid stabilization and blocking receptor binding. A12 binds the site at the bottom of the canyon surrounding the 5-fold vertex, while all VHHs bind at or near the quasi-3-fold vertex, where these sites extensively overlap with the CD155-binding sites (Table 1). For EV-D68, a member of human type D enterovirus (HEV-D), sialic acid [54, 55] and intercellular adhesion molecule 5 (ICAM-5) [56] have been identified as its functional receptors. Sialic acid has been reported to bind into the viral canyon region [54], whereas the binding site of ICAM-5 remains unclear. Three antibodies (228 [57], 159 [57] and 8F12 [58]) appear capable of inhibiting EV-D68 attachment to cell surface. The 8F12-binding footprints and the binding sites of human antibodies 228 and 159 are partially in or adjacent to the canyon-binding site, thus explaining the experiment observation that these antibodies could inhibit the binding of EV-D68 to the sialic acid receptor. Moreover, several nAbs have been reported to target regions that are distant from the known receptor binding sites, including E19 [59] against EV-A71, 1D5 [60] against CV-A6, C3 [61] against PV-1 and 11G1 [62] against EV-D68 (Table 1). These antibodies might neutralize the virus by preventing binding to unidentified cellular receptors or stabilizing the viral capsid in a unique binding manner. For example, C3 binds bivalently to poliovirus at the 5-fold vertex, and that binding may inhibit the formation of a transient state [61]. In contrast, 11G1 exclusively recognizes the A-particle of EV-D68 at the 5-fold vertex. It binds two adjacent protomers from neighboring VP1 proteins, suggesting that 11G1 neutralizes with assistance from other factors and potentially achieves neutralization by interfering with genome release from the A-particles into host cells [62].

Inducing Conformational Changes of Virions via Functional Mimicry

Enterovirus infection begins with the attachment of a mature virion to attachment and uncoating receptors, followed by the transformation of the virion into a cell-entry intermediate known as the A-particle. This transformation results in the release of the viral genome into the host cell's cytosol. Throughout the lifecycle, enteroviruses undergo structural transitions of their capsids, observing four primary particle forms: procapsid, mature virion, A-particle and empty particle [1]. These variations in particle forms play a critical role in viral infection. Notably, neutralizing antibodies against enteroviruses have been found to induce capsid destabilization, mimicking the function of uncoating receptors and triggering conformational changes to varying degrees. Nanobodies known as VHHs that specifically recognize poliovirus type 1 have previously been identified as potential antiviral agents [53]. The VHHs, specifically PVSS21E, bind deep within the virus canyon at sites that extensively overlap with the binding site for the receptor (CD155) [53]. This binding of PVSS21E leads to significant changes in the structure of the capsid, ultimately trapping the virus in an early expansion stage. Notably, the binding of PVSS21E induces significant alterations on the top surface of VP1, impacting the B and C beta strands, the BC and DE loops and the CD helix (Table 1). However, most of the remaining VP1 beta barrel remains largely unaffected. Notably, the changes resulting from PVSS21E binding can be accommodated by the conformational changes of the pocket factor, which remains bound. These changes are less drastic than the structural modifications induced by receptor binding, which significantly block the pocket, expelling the pocket factor and preventing its reattachment. Overall, the PVSS21E-poliovirus complex offers insights into the early stages of the particle expansion process. It can be conceptualized as a reversible and early stage in the expansion process, with a delicate balance between the stabilizing effect of PVSS21E (which blocks infection) and the destabilization of the virus associated with the structural changes necessary for expansion. PVSS21E binding establishes stabilizing contacts within regions that change expansion and prevent the release of the pocket factor.

Furthermore, similar to the observations on poliovirus, our previous study reported that an EV-D68-specific neutralizing antibody, named 15C5, binds and triggers the transformation of mature virions into classical A-particles, thus mimicking host receptor interactions [62]. When 15C5 binds mature virions at the 3-fold axes, it leads to the separation of the VP2 HI loop and the VP3 BC loop, initiating a conformational change from mature virion to A-particle through a cascade of molecular rearrangements and allosteric effects (Table 1). 15C5 demonstrates the ability to bind to all variations of the virions, allowing it to not only induce viral conformational change to A-particles but also inhibit the attachment of A-particles to cell surface receptors, resulting in the neutralization of viral infection. Analysis based on the structure of the binding process reveals that 15C5 recognizes a quaternary epitope spanning across VP3 and the VP2 of two adjacent protomers. This interaction potentially restricts the capsid at an intermediate stage, impeding further conformational changes and the uncoating process. Additionally, a preliminary study indicated that the antigen-binding fragment of a neutralizing antibody, C5, binds to the neutralizing immunogenic (NIm)-III site by making contact with a closely located area on the outer surface of human Rhinovirus B14 (HRV-B14) [63]. This interaction leads to notable structural changes in the capsid, facilitating the release of the viral genome. The process of C5-induced virus uncoating is influenced by temperature and the ratio of the virus to Fab. Notably, this neutralization mechanism differs from antibodies PVSS21E and 15C5 against poliovirus and EV-D68, in which antibodies do not appear to induce premature viral uncoating and genome release. Moreover, an interesting finding is that 2H12-mediated neutralization of EV-D68 can also trigger virus uncoating [58]. In comparison with PVSS21E, 15C5, and C5, 2H12 was found to impair EV-D68 viral particles to some extent, induce capsid expansion to form three distinct conformational states and cause premature release of a portion of viral RNA from the capsid, probably leading to decreased viral infectivity. It is worth noting that the aforementioned antibodies bind to regions surrounding the three-fold axes or near the quasi-3-fold vertex of the viral capsid and across the interface between protomers. However, for 2H12, its binding site lies near the canyon and around the two-fold axes, suggesting 2H12 may use a distinct mechanism to induce virus uncoating.

Destabilizing the Capsid and Inducing Virion Disruption

In addition to the well-established mechanisms of action, specific antibodies have demonstrated an ability to act through kinetic mechanisms involving the facilitated dissociation of targeted complexes [64-66]. Facilitated dissociation refers to the process in which "disruptive" inhibitors engage targets that are sequestered in stable macromolecular complexes, accelerate their dissociation and subsequently inactivate them. This mechanism differs from simply blocking protein interactions. Structural studies have shown that disruptive inhibitors and pairs of antibodies that can displace each other mediate disruption through small regions of predicted steric conflict, in contrast to competitive inhibitors that exhibit large regions of steric conflict. For example, Huo et al. discovered that the antibody CR3022 exhibits strong affinity to the receptor binding domain (RBD) of the SARS-CoV-2 spike protein at a distinct site from the receptor's binding site [67]. Furthermore, the antibody CR3022 effectively neutralizes the virus, as cryo-EM analysis illustrates its capability to disrupt the spike protein. On the other hand, physical collisions at the molecular level frequently lead to significant structural and conformational modifications in protein ensembles composed of multiple subunits [68]. Previous studies have demonstrated that physical disturbances can influence virus dissociation under in vitro conditions. Research on hepatitis E virus (HEV) has revealed that nAb 8C11 binding is located near the protrusion spike of the HEV virus-like particles (VLPs) [69]. It causes significant physical collisions between the antibody and the capsid, dissociating VLPs into homodimer species within two hours.

Table 1. Summary of neutralizing antibodies against human enteroviruses according to their antiviral mechanism

Neutralizing mechanism	Antigen	Antibody	Immunogen/ Source	Potency *in vitro*	Potency *in vivo**	Major binding sites	Reference
Capsid stabilization							
Targeting/partially targeting/adjacent to the known receptor binding domains							
	EV-A71	MA28-7	EV-A71 particle	Highest neutralizing titer: 1350	-	5-fold vertex; VP1 BC-loop (E98), VP1 DE-loop (Q145), VP1 HI-loop (K242, K244)	Lee et al. (2013) [39]
		22A12	SP55 and SP70	Neutralizing titer: 16	-	Canyon region; VP1 GH-loop (K215, E217, K218, D219)	Li et al. (2009) [32], Shingler et al. (2015) [33]
		D5	EV-A71 VLP	IC_{50}: 0.183-1.592 μg/mL	100% (10 μg/g, 6-day-old ICR mice)	2-fold vertex; VP1 GH-loop (T210, K215-L220), VP2 βD-sheet (Y100), VP2 EF-loop (E142, D143, P147, Y148), VP3 CD-loop (R87, R92), VP3 EF-loop (G139-P141), VP3 GH-loop (R182, D187)	Ku et al. (2012) [90], Ku et al. (2015) [91], Ye et al., (2016) [34]
		D6	EV-A71 E- and F-particles	IC_{50}: 1 nM	-	3-fold vertex; VP3 "puff," VP3 BC-loop, VP2 GH-loop, VP1 C-terminus (A280-T292)	Zhu et al. (2018) [35]
		38-1-10A	An EV-A71-infected child	IC_{50}: 0.047-13.17 μg/mL	100% (10 μg/g, hSCRAB2-transgenic C57BL/6 mice)	3-fold vertex; VP2 HI-loop, VP2 BC-loop (S75–G77), VP3 HI-loop (N210)	Huang et al. (2020) [36]
		38-3-11A		IC_{50}: 0.007-2.568 μg/mL	-	3-fold vertex; VP2 HI-loop, VP3 BC-loop, VP3 HI-loop	
		E1	EV-A71-infected patients	IC_{50}: 0.195-0.78 μg/mL, can not neutralized BrCr(A) strain	100% (10 μg/g, 10- or 11-day-old BALB/c mice)**	5-fold vertex; VP1 BC-loop (P96-N102), VP1 HI-loop (G239-L247)	Chen et al. (2022) [40]

Table 1. (Continued)

Neutralizing mechanism	Antigen	Antibody	Immunogen/ Source	Potency *in vitro*	Potency *in vivo**	Major binding sites	Reference
	CV-A16	NA9D7	CV-A16 cell culture	IC_{50}: 0.51-1.96 μg/mL	100% (3 μg/g, one-day-old BALB/c mice)	2-fold vertex; VP1 GH-loop (E213-Q224), VP2 EF-loop (E142-H145), VP3 GH-loop (R182-D187)	Ye et al. (2016) [92], He et al. (2020) [37]
		14B10		IC_{50}: 0.23-1.04 μg/mL	100% (3 μg/g, one-day-old BALB/c mice)	3-fold vertex; VP2 BC-loop (K69-W78), VP2 EF-loop (Q155-V159), VP2 HI-loop (G227-E231), VP3 BC-loop (V75-K78)	
		18A7		IC_{50}: 0.04-0.13 μg/mL, can not neutralized 4479(A) strain	no protection (even at a 30 μg/g dosage)	5-fold vertex; VP1 BC-loop (P96), VP1 DE-loop (K141-P148), VP1 HI-loop (E241-S246)	
		9B5	CV-A16 particle	IC_{50}: 0.0004-0.0024 μg/mL	100% (10 μg/g, 2-day-old ICR mice)	5-fold vertex; VP1 BC-loop (G99 and D104), VP1 EF-loop (R166), VP1 HI-loop (K242)	Zhang et al. (2022) [38]
		8C4		IC_{50}: 0.052-0.074 μg/mL	91.7%-100% (10 μg/g, 2-day-old ICR mice)	3-fold vertex; VP3 BC-loop (S77), VP3 HI-loop (T210), VP2 HI-loop (G227, A228, S230, E231), VP2 βB-sheet (K69), VP2 βC-sheet (W78), VP2 BC-loop (D74)	
	CV-A10	2G8	CV-A10 mature virion	IC_{50}: 0.2 μg/mL	100% (30 μg/g, one-day-old BALB/c mice)	quasi-3-fold vertex; VP1 C-terminus (D279-I283, D289), VP2 EF-loop (R135, Y162, D163), VP3 AB-loop (T58, E60, T62)	Zhu et al. (2018) [43]
	CV-B1	2E6	CV-B1 particle	IC_{50}: 0.152 μg/mL	100% (1 μg/g, one-day-old BALB/c mice)	3-fold vertex; VP2 BC-loop (M72, N74), VP2 EF-loop (S144, E145, R153, M154, T156-A165, K167)	Zheng et al. (2022) [45]

Neutralizing mechanism	Antigen	Antibody	Immunogen/ Source	Potency *in vitro*	Potency *in vivo**	Major binding sites	Reference
	CV-B1	8A10		IC_{50}: 0.012 μg/mL	100% (0.1 μg/g, one-day-old BALB/c mice)	5-fold vertex; VP1 βD-sheet (Q125), VP1 EF-loop (K155), VP1 GH-loop (K230), VP1 HI-loop (Q254, E256, K257, P265-G267), VP2 EF-loop (N136-N138, Q159, G161-S163), VP3 BC-loop (E59, D60, S63), VP3 C-terminus (R232, D234-Q238)	
	CV-B1	9A3		IC_{50}: 0.376 μg/mL	100% (1 μg/g, one-day-old BALB/c mice)	quasi-3-fold vertex; VP2 EF-loop (M72, N74, M154, T156-Q159, G161, S163, N164), VP3 BC-loop (E59, D60, S63, S64, K66)	
	E30	6C5	E30 mature virion	IC_{50}: 1.2 nM	-	5-fold vertex; VP1 BC-loop (E82-V84, D86, E87, D89, Y91), VP1 DE-loop (T130), VP1 EF-loop (K156, E159), VP1 HI-loop (T229)	Wang et al. (2020) [49]
	E30	4B10		IC_{50}: 0.3 nM	-	Canyon region; VP2 EF-loop (T137, D138, K159, T161, T163), VP1 C-terminus (L260 and N268), VP3 C-terminus (Q234)	
	E3	5G3	E3 F-particle	IC_{50}: 0.34 nM	-	2-fold vertex; VP1 C-terminus (T283-V287, H292), VP3 EF-loop (S140, Q143)	Feng et al. (2021) [50]
	E3	6D10		IC_{50}: 0.65 nM	-	2-fold vertex; VP1 C-terminus (L284, P286, V287, Y289, H292), VP3 EF-loop (S140, Q143)	Qi et al. (2022) [51]
	PV-1/ PV-2	A12	PV-immunized chimpanzees	Highest neutralizing titer: 1722, can not neutralized PV-3 starin	-	5-fold vertex; VP1 BC-loop (V107, W108), VP1 GH-loop (A223, L234), VP1 C-terminus (S295), VP2 EF-loop (T167, T168), VP3 CD-loop (S91-P93)	Chen et al. (2011 [93], 2013 [52])
	PV-1	PVSP29F PVSP19B PVSP6A PVSS8A	A PV-1-immunized dromedary	neutralizing VHHs	-	quasi-3-fold vertex; a portion of the VP2 EF-loop (around T138-H142), VP1 GH-loop (Y209-F237), VP1 EF-loop (V160-N180), VP1 Cβ-sheet (and vicinity; D102-T115), VP1 C-terminal (near Y280)	Strauss et al. (2016) [53]

Table 1. (Continued)

Neutralizing mechanism	Antigen	Antibody	Immunogen/ Source	Potency *in vitro*	Potency *in vivo**	Major binding sites	Reference
	EV-D68	228	12 EV-D68-infected participants	IC_{50}: 0.0037-0.052 μg/mL	100% (10 μg/g, ten-day-old AG129 mice)	5-fold vertex; VP1 βB-sheet (K71-S73), VP1 DE-loop (G129), VP1 C-terminus (K268), VP2 EF-loop (N136), VP3 C-terminus (G234, L236-H238, E243)	Vogt et al. (2020) [57]
		159		IC_{50}: 0.00032-38 μg/mL, can not neutralized KY/53(D) strain	-	3-fold vertex; VP1 C-terminus (E271, R272, D285), VP3 N-terminus (S60, M64, E65)	
		8F12	EVD68 VLP	IC_{50}: 0.49-125 μg/mL	100% (10 μg/g, one-day-old ICR mice)	Canyon region; VP2 EF-loop (N136, T139, S140), VP1 GH-loop (N206), VP1 BC-loop (R85), VP3 C-terminus (A244)	Zhang et al. (2021) [58]
Far from the known receptor binding domain							
	EV-A71	E19	EV-A71 E-particle	IC_{50}: >0.1 nM	-	3-fold vertex; VP3 "knob"	Plevka et al. (2014) [59]
	CV-A6	1D5	CV-A6 cell culture	IC_{50}: 0.94 μg/mL	-	5-fold vertex; VP1 BC-loop (T96-D99), VP1 EF-loop (D159-K162, Y164), VP1 HI-loop (S236, T237, G239), VP1 DE-loop (N138)	Xu et al. (2017) [60]
	PV-1	C3	PV-1 80S particle	neutralizing mAb	-	5-fold vertex; VP1 BC-loop (D93-K103)	Lin et al. (2013) [61]
	EV-D68	11G1	EV-D68 cell culture	IC_{50}: 39.7 μg/mL	Reduced illness severity and delayed mortality (60 μg/g, one-day-old BALB/c mice)	5-fold vertex; VP1 βB-sheet (E75), VP1 BC-loop (T80-S82, A84, D87), VP1 EF-loop (K157), VP1 βI-sheet (T234)	Zheng et al. (2018) [62]

Neutralizing mechanism	Antigen	Antibody	Immunogen/ Source	Potency *in vitro*	Potency *in vivo**	Major binding sites	Reference
Triggered capsid conformational changes and/or genome release							
	HRV-B14	C5	-	neutralizing mAb	-	3-fold vertex; VP1 C-terminus (K281, D285, K287), VP2 C-terminus (P227-T229), VP3 N-terminus (T58-T60), VP3 BC-loop (N72, N74-Q76, E78), VP3 HI-loop (T202-Q204, Y206)	Dong et al. (2017) [63]
	PV-1	PVSS21E	A PV-1-immunized dromedary	neutralizing VHHs	-	quasi-3-fold vertex; a portion of the VP2 EF-loop (around T138-H142), VP1 GH-loop (Y209-F237), VP1 EF-loop (V160-N180), VP1 Cβ-sheet (and vicinity; D102-T115), VP1 C-terminal (near Y280)	Strauss et al. (2016) [53]
	EV-D68	15C5	EV-D68 cell culture	IC_{50}: 1.5 μg/mL	100% (60 μg/g, one-day-old BALB/c mice)	3-fold vertex; VP2 BC-loop (K67, K70, E72, S75), VP3 AB-loop (S60), VP3 BC-loop (S72, D76), VP3 HI-loop (D208)	Zheng et al. (2018) [62]
		2H12	EV-D68 VLP	IC_{50}: 0.12-1.95 μg/mL, can not neutralized Fermon (prototype) strain	100% (10 μg/g, one-day-old ICR mice)	Canyon region; VP1 GH-loop (K205, N206), VP2 EF-loop (H135, N136, N138-S140, D144, D145, H157), VP3 C-terminus (H240, A244, Q247)	Zhang et al. (2021) [58]
Capsid destablization and virion disruption							
	EV-A71	E18	EV-A71 E-particle	IC_{50}: >0.1 nM	-	3-fold vertex; VP2 EF-loop (K149)	Plevka et al. (2014) [59]
		A9	EV-A71 E- and F-particles	IC_{50}: 0.1 nM	-	3-fold vertex; VP3 "puff," VP3-BC loop, VP3 α2-helix (K144-M150), VP1 C-terminus (A289-I294)	Zhu et al. (2018) [35]
	CV-B1	5F5	CV-B1 mature virion	IC_{50}: 0.11-1.49 μg/mL	100% (1 μg/g, one-day-old BALB/c mice)	3-fold vertex; VP2 BC-loop (E67, V69, Q70, M72, N74), VP2 EF-loop (S144, E145, M154, S163, N164, K167), VP2 HI-loop (Y233, S237, P239, Y240), VP3 BC-loop (Q73, S74, S76, N78), VP3 HI-loop (V200)	Xu et al. (2021) [70]

-, No data; *, Antibodies administered at 24 hour-post infection; **, Antibodies administered at 12 hour-post infection.

In enteroviruses, some neutralizing antibodies utilize an antibody-mediated disruption mechanism to exert their neutralizing activity (Table 1). The highly potent neutralizing antibody, named A9, can destabilize EV-A71 virions to induce genome release and damage EV-A71 particles to some extent at physiological temperatures [35]. The footprint of the A9 spanned the region between the 2-fold and the 3-fold axes, including VP3 "puff," the VP3 BC loop, VP3 α2 and the VP1 C terminus (Table 1). This binding region is broadly similar in location to the previously observed E18 bound to EV-A71 [59]. Notably, our team shows evidence of a vigorous mode of antibody-mediated disruption induced by the physical disruption of the CV-B1. We have screened for neutralizing antibodies by performing a CAR-based competitive binding assay. The discovery of CAR-guided led to a potent therapeutic antibody, 5F5, which neutralizes viral infection by interfering with CAR-virion interactions [70]. Intriguingly, 5F5 binding causes capsid changes, including receptor-initiated capsid destabilization, conformational changes on the VP2 EF loop, and viral disruption (Table 1). The binding of 5F5 to the mature virion leads to two competing consequences: viral capsid destabilization, which results in the forming of a metastable A-particle, and blockage of structural transformation. These consequences may ultimately cause viral dissociation. In contrast to A9 against EV-A71, 5F5 destabilizes and, to some extent, disrupts the virus at room temperature before the virus can enter host cells [35]. Less-violent inhibition mechanisms, such as destabilizing the virion structure and initiating the release of viral genomes, are commonly observed in picornaviruses through neutralizing antibodies. Examples of such antibodies include E18 (anti-EV-A71) [59] and R10 (anti-hepatitis A virus) [71], which mimic cell receptors. The destabilization and disruption of viral particles by nAbs predominantly occur in regions adjacent to the icosahedral 2-fold axes, which separate during the initial stage of uncoating in enteroviruses [72, 73]. These results should inform the rational design of novel therapeutic countermeasures against diseases caused by CVB and other picornaviruses.

Fc-Dependent Effector Functions

Antiviral antibodies of the IgG class are often bi-functional. Antibodies' antigen binding domain (Fab) can directly neutralize viral infectivity. In addition, upon Fab-mediated binding to viral antigens on the surface of infected cells, the antibody's crystallizable fragment (Fc) can contribute significantly to their in vivo efficacy. The binding of FcγRs to effector cells can lead to complement-dependent cytotoxicity, antibody-dependent cellular cytotoxicity (ADCC), and antibody-dependent cellular phagocytosis (ADCP) [74]. Indeed, there are several instances in which highly effective neutralizing mAbs lose their ability to provide antiviral protection in vivo when interactions between Fc and FcγR are disrupted. Conversely, antibodies with non-neutralizing/weakly neutralizing activity in vitro assays can still confer strong antiviral protection in vivo, indicating that these antibodies' effectiveness relies on engaging FcγR activation.

Previous studies have identified similar cases in which non-neutralizing antibodies provide protection against SARS-CoV-2, West Nile Virus (WNV) and alphaviruses [75-77]. For instance, recent studies have demonstrated that the Fc effector functions are crucial in providing optimal protection through mAb therapy against SARS-CoV-2 [77]. Intact mAbs, when administered after infection, showed superior efficacy in reducing the burden of SARS-CoV-2 and lung disease in animals compared to loss-of-function Fc variant mAbs. These effects were attributed to the ability of intact mAbs to mitigate inflammation and improve respiratory mechanics. However, enterovirus vaccine evaluation prioritizes neutralizing antibodies while neglecting the significance of non-neutralizing/weak antibodies. While developing enterovirus vaccines, manufacturers have observed that antibodies generated by the vaccine, despite having low neutralizing titers, still demonstrate protective effects in animals. Previous research has found that a potential preventive and therapeutic effect could be mediated by a non-neutralizing antibody targeting the VP2 EF loop of CV-A16 via the Fc-dependent effector mechanism [78]. These findings shed light on the previously unexplored protective role of non-neutralizing antibodies in viral infections and offer new insights for developing and assessing vaccines. Therefore, non-neutralizing/weak antibodies should be given more attention in the surveillance of epidemic and enterovirus vaccine development and evaluation.

Structural Basis for the Synergistic Neutralization

Neutralizing antibody cocktails are promising therapeutic agents that can be used for better prevention and treatment of viral infectious diseases. For example, REGN-COV2 is a cocktail of two highly effective neutralizing antibodies that target distinct epitopes of the SARS-CoV-2 virus [79, 80]. This cocktail has demonstrated the ability to significantly reduce the viral load and is currently undergoing clinical trials. ZMappTM is a three-antibody cocktail targeting the Ebola glycoprotein [81]. It has proven one of the most successful antibody-based therapeutics for treating Ebola virus infections. Furthermore, developing two-antibody cocktails that target the canyon region of the mature virion has shown adequate protection against EV-D68 in animal models [58]. Recently, we have systematically investigated the molecular basis of potent and synergistic neutralization mediated by two- or three-antibody cocktails against CVB1 [45]. Through cryo-EM structure analysis, we observed that the two-antibody cocktails (8A10/C2E6 or 8A10/C9A3) bound to distinct viral particle types, with a total of three or four different kinds of nAbs interacting. Specifically, 8A10 is preferentially bound to mature virions and pre-A particles, while 2E6 and 9A3 are bound to A-particles and empty particles, respectively. This binding pattern revealed that the two-antibody cocktails induce conformational changes in CVB1 mature virions by coordinated binding to different conformational states, resulting in synergistic neutralization against CVB1. In contrast, the three-antibody cocktail (8A10/2E6/9A3) demonstrated highly efficient viral uncoating and even disrupted CVB1 virions. Notably, the mechanism of neutralization mediated by this cocktail differs from other reported cocktail therapies targeting nonoverlapping epitopes on viral glycoproteins, as seen in SARS-CoV-2 or Ebolavirus cases.

Typically, a rational design of therapeutic mAb cocktails aims to prevent escape mutations while maximizing the occupancy of antibodies on the virion by minimizing steric interference between mAbs, thereby requiring the selection of non-competing mAbs. However, our elegant demonstration indicates that this approach may overlook potential synergistic mAb combinations that exhibit high efficacy in vivo. The field faces the challenge of further developing empirical approaches to identify synergistic mAb combinations, instead of solely relying on conventional wisdom.

Conclusion and Future Perspectives

Enterovirus infection can cause a variety of diseases, including HFMD, non-specific febrile illness, neonatal sepsis-like disease, encephalitis, paralysis and respiratory diseases. Enteroviruses display complex epidemiological characteristics with frequent co-circulation patterns among serotypes [82]. This highlights the necessity for therapeutic agents with broad effectiveness. Different types of enteroviruses have similar processes of uncoating and RNA release, suggesting the presence of conserved intermediate conformation domains that may serve as ideal targets for discovering broad-spectrum antiviral epitopes. Enteroviruses invade target cells through different receptors and endocytic pathways. Upon entry, they may utilize common mechanisms to release their RNA genome, which involves interactions between the viral capsid, receptors, acidic conditions of endosomes and endosomal membrane. For example, VP4 has shown the ability to insert into the lipid bilayer, forming membrane pores [83]. At the same time, the conserved N-terminal region of VP1 acts as a dual-function transmembrane anchor, facilitating the localization of the intermediate particle to the membrane and enabling the release of the viral genome [19, 84]. Previous studies have found that the host factor phospholipase A2 group XVI (PLA2G16) is a standard host factor for enteroviruses, promoting the translocation of viral genomes within endosomes containing the virus [85]. PLA2G16 is believed to be involved in the formation, expansion, or maintenance of membrane pores. It mediates the release of viral genomes by directly interacting with enterovirus proteins or nucleic acids. Although PLA2G16 receptor has been identified, the exact mechanism by which PLA2G16 mediate infection is still poorly understood. Further studies are necessary to improve our understanding of virus infection and pathogenesis and define new intervention targets. Advanced microscopy techniques are increasingly accessible, such as three-dimensional scanning electron microscopy (3D SEM) approaches which enable the reconstruction of entire cells and visualization of virus-induced intracellular changes. Additionally, in situ, cryo-electron tomography, an imaging technique that enables the structural analysis of macromolecular complexes within their physiological microenvironment, can provide valuable insights into viral replication complexes and their association with replication organelles.

More extraordinary efforts should be devoted to developing preventive and therapeutic options for controlling enterovirus infections. With new understandings of the viral life cycle and advancements in computational drug discovery, the development of innovative and comprehensive enterovirus inhibitors is anticipated. Aside from pocket factor analogs that stabilize the virion, molecules targeting viral proteins or host factors involved in pore formation and capable of preventing genome translocation may serve as broadly promising candidates [86, 87]. To complete the infection and transition from mature virions to empty particles, enteroviruses might have certain hidden domains within the capsid, such as receptor-binding domains and the N-termini of VP4 and VP1, which interact with host cells. These domains are highly conserved among different subtypes and might be ideal targets for discovering broad-spectrum antiviral epitopes. PLA2G16, the pan-enterovirus host factor is necessary for the replication of all tested enteroviruses. Because no selective inhibitors targeting PLA2G16 have been reported thus far, developing rapid and reliable strategies to isolate these antibodies, particularly broadly potent neutralizing antibodies, is crucial for enhancing the response to enterovirus and better preparing for emergent infectious diseases in the future. For example, nanobodies, found exclusively in camelids and cartilaginous fish like sharks, comprise a unique class of antibodies characterized by a single variable heavy chain region (VHH) and the absence of CH2 and CH3 regions, resulting in a naturally occurring light chain deficiency [88]. This structural difference imparts hydrophilicity to nanobodies, making them small and remarkably stable even under extreme temperatures or pH conditions. Despite being only a tenth of the molecular weight of conventional antibodies, the VHH region maintains complete antigenic specificity at approximately 15 kDa [89]. This distinctive trait allows nanobodies to access epitopes typically inaccessible to traditional antibodies, including conserved and hidden domains [88]. Moreover, nanobodies can be genetically engineered into bifunctional or bispecific antibodies for precise targeting in disease intervention. The genetic modification of nanobodies to form polymers notably enhances their antigen-binding capabilities. Additionally, emerging and re-emerging enteroviruses pose a severe threat to public health. Intensified efforts should be undertaken to explore the possibility of combining multiple mAbs that recognize distinct viral sites into a diverse antibody cocktail to bolster the therapeutic response against the constantly mutating viral landscape.

Acknowledgments

This work was supported by grants from the National Natural Science Foundation of China (No. 82172248, 82101918 and 82272310), the China Postdoctoral Science Foundation (No. 2022T150550).

Competing Interests

The authors declare no potential conflicts of interest.

References

[1] Baggen J, Thibaut H J, Strating J, et al. The life cycle of non-polio enteroviruses and how to target it. *Nat Rev Microbiol*, 2018, 16(6): 368-381.

[2] Cox B, Levent F. Hand, Foot, and Mouth Disease. *JAMA*, 2018, 320(23): 2492.

[3] Kennedy J L, Turner R B, Braciale T, et al. Pathogenesis of rhinovirus infection. *Curr Opin Virol*, 2012, 2(3): 287-93.

[4] Uprety P, Graf E H. Enterovirus infection and acute flaccid myelitis. *Curr Opin Virol*, 2020, 40: 55-60.

[5] Messacar K, Asturias E J, Hixon A M, et al. Enterovirus D68 and acute flaccid myelitis-evaluating the evidence for causality. *Lancet Infect Dis*, 2018, 18(8): e239-e247.

[6] Hasbun R, Rosenthal N, Balada-Llasat J M, et al. Epidemiology of Meningitis and Encephalitis in the United States, 2011-2014. *Clin Infect Dis*, 2017, 65(3): 359-363.

[7] Hasbun R, Wootton S H, Rosenthal N, et al. Epidemiology of Meningitis and Encephalitis in Infants and Children in the United States, 2011-2014. *Pediatr Infect Dis J*, 2019, 38(1): 37-41.

[8] Daba T M, Zhao Y, Pan Z. Advancement of Mechanisms of Coxsackie Virus B3-Induced Myocarditis Pathogenesis and the Potential Therapeutic Targets. *Curr Drug Targets*, 2019, 20(14): 1461-1473.

[9] Hober D, Alidjinou E K. Diabetes: Towards a coxsackievirus B-based vaccine to combat T1DM. *Nat Rev Endocrinol*, 2018, 14(3): 131-132.

[10] Cafferkey J, Coultas J A, Mallia P. Human rhinovirus infection and COPD: role in exacerbations and potential for therapeutic targets. *Expert Rev Respir Med*, 2020, 14(8): 777-789.

[11] Ortega H, Nickle D, Carter L. Rhinovirus and asthma: Challenges and opportunities. *Rev Med Virol*, 2021, 31(4): e2193.

[12] Zhu F C, Xu W B, Xia J L, et al. Efficacy, Safety, and Immunogenicity of an Enterovirus 71 Vaccine in China. *New England Journal of Medicine*, 2014, 370(9): 818-828.

[13] Li R C, Liu L D, Mo Z J, et al. An Inactivated Enterovirus 71 Vaccine in Healthy Children. *New England Journal of Medicine*, 2014, 370(9): 829-837.

[14] Zhu F C, Meng F Y, Li J X, et al. Efficacy, safety, and immunology of an inactivated alum-adjuvant enterovirus 71 vaccine in children in China: a multicentre, randomised, double-blind, placebo-controlled, phase 3 trial. *Lancet*, 2013, 381(9882): 2024-2032.

[15] Plevka P, Perera R, Cardosa J, et al. Crystal structure of human enterovirus 71. *Science*, 2012, 336(6086): 1274.

[16] Rossmann M G, Arnold E, Erickson J W, et al. Structure of a human common cold virus and functional relationship to other picornaviruses. *Nature*, 1985, 317(6033): 145-53.

[17] Baggen J, Hurdiss D L, Zocher G, et al. Role of enhanced receptor engagement in the evolution of a pandemic acute hemorrhagic conjunctivitis virus. *Proceedings of the National Academy of Sciences of the United States of America*, 2018, 115(2): 397-402.

[18] Li Q, Yafal A G, Lee Y M, et al. Poliovirus neutralization by antibodies to internal epitopes of VP4 and VP1 results from reversible exposure of these sequences at physiological temperature. *J Virol*, 1994, 68(6): 3965-70.

[19] Fricks C E, Hogle J M. Cell-induced conformational change in poliovirus: externalization of the amino terminus of VP1 is responsible for liposome binding. *J Virol*, 1990, 64(5): 1934-45.

[20] Shingler K L, Yoder J L, Carnegie M S, et al. The enterovirus 71 A-particle forms a gateway to allow genome release: a cryoEM study of picornavirus uncoating. *PLoS Pathog*, 2013, 9(3): e1003240.

[21] Levy H C, Bostina M, Filman D J, et al. Catching a virus in the act of RNA release: a novel poliovirus uncoating intermediate characterized by cryo-electron microscopy. *J Virol*, 2010, 84(9): 4426-41.

[22] Pickl-Herk A, Luque D, Vives-Adrián L, et al. Uncoating of common cold virus is preceded by RNA switching as determined by X-ray and cryo-EM analyses of the subviral A-particle. *Proceedings of the National Academy of Sciences of the United States of America*, 2013, 110(50): 20063-20068.

[23] Chang L Y, King C C, Hsu K H, et al. Risk factors of enterovirus 71 infection and associated hand, foot, and mouth disease/herpangina in children during an epidemic in Taiwan. *Pediatrics*, 2002, 109(6): e88.

[24] Jin P, Li J, Zhang X, et al. Validation and evaluation of serological correlates of protection for inactivated enterovirus 71 vaccine in children aged 6-35 months. Hum *Vaccin Immunother*, 2016, 12(4): 916-21.

[25] Yamayoshi S, Yamashita Y, Li J F, et al. Scavenger receptor B2 is a cellular receptor for enterovirus 71. *Nature Medicine*, 2009, 15(7): 798-U15.

[26] Yamayoshi S, Iizuka S, Yamashita T, et al. Human SCARB2-Dependent Infection by Coxsackievirus A7, A14, and A16 and Enterovirus 71. *Journal of Virology*, 2012, 86(10): 5686-5696.

[27] Nishimura Y, Shimojima M, Tano Y, et al. Human P-selectin glycoprotein ligand-1 is a functional receptor for enterovirus 71. *Nature Medicine*, 2009, 15(7): 794-U14.

[28] Nishimura Y, Shimizu H. Cellular receptors for human enterovirus species a. *Front Microbiol*, 2012, 3: 105.

[29] Yamayoshi S, Fujii K, Koike S. Receptors for enterovirus 71. *Emerg Microbes Infect*, 2014, 3(7): e53.

[30] Zhang X, Shi J, Ye X, et al. Coxsackievirus A16 utilizes cell surface heparan sulfate glycosaminoglycans as its attachment receptor. *Emerg Microbes Infect*, 2017, 6(7): e65.

[31] Zhou D M, Zhao Y G, Kotecha A, et al. Unexpected mode of engagement between enterovirus 71 and its receptor SCARB2. *Nature Microbiology*, 2019, 4(3): 414-419.

[32] Li X, Mao C, Ma S, et al. Generation of neutralizing monoclonal antibodies against Enterovirus 71 using synthetic peptides. *Biochem Biophys Res Commun*, 2009, 390(4): 1126-8.

[33] Shingler K L, Cifuente J O, Ashley R E, et al. The Enterovirus 71 Procapsid Binds Neutralizing Antibodies and Rescues Virus Infection In Vitro. *Journal of Virology*, 2015, 89(3): 1900-1908.

[34] Ye X, Fan C, Ku Z, et al. Structural Basis for Recognition of Human Enterovirus 71 by a Bivalent Broadly Neutralizing Monoclonal Antibody. *PLoS Pathog*, 2016, 12(3): e1005454.

[35] Zhu L, Xu K, Wang N, et al. Neutralization Mechanisms of Two Highly Potent Antibodies against Human Enterovirus 71. *mBio*, 2018, 9(4).

[36] Huang K A, Zhou D, Fry E E, et al. Structural and functional analysis of protective antibodies targeting the threefold plateau of enterovirus 71. *Nat Commun*, 2020, 11(1): 5253.

[37] He M Z, Xu L F, Zheng Q B, et al. Identification of Antibodies with Non-overlapping Neutralization Sites that Target Coxsackievirus A16. *Cell Host & Microbe*, 2020, 27(2): 249-261.

[38] Zhang C, Liu C, Shi J, et al. Molecular mechanism of antibody neutralization of coxsackievirus A16. *Nat Commun*, 2022, 13(1): 7854.

[39] Lee H, Cifuente J O, Ashley R E, et al. A strain-specific epitope of enterovirus 71 identified by cryo-electron microscopy of the complex with fab from neutralizing antibody. *J Virol*, 2013, 87(21): 11363-70.

[40] Chen Z, Bao L, Zhu B, et al. Structural and functional analysis of a potent human neutralizing antibody against enterovirus A71. *Sci China Life Sci*, 2022, 65(12): 2517-2526.

[41] Staring J, Van Den Hengel L G, Raaben M, et al. KREMEN1 Is a Host Entry Receptor for a Major Group of Enteroviruses. *Cell Host & Microbe*, 2018, 23(5): 636-+.

[42] Zhao Y G, Zhou D M, Ni T, et al. Hand-foot-and-mouth disease virus receptor KREMEN1 binds the canyon of Coxsackie Virus A10. *Nature Communications*, 2020, 11(1).

[43] Zhu R, Xu L, Zheng Q, et al. Discovery and structural characterization of a therapeutic antibody against coxsackievirus A10. *Sci Adv*, 2018, 4(9): eaat7459.

[44] Bergelson J M, Cunningham J A, Droguett G, et al. Isolation of a common receptor for Coxsackie B viruses and adenoviruses 2 and 5. *Science*, 1997, 275(5304): 1320-3.

[45] Zheng Q, Zhu R, Yin Z, et al. Structural basis for the synergistic neutralization of coxsackievirus B1 by a triple-antibody cocktail. *Cell Host Microbe*, 2022, 30(9): 1279-1294 e6.

[46] Bergelson J M, Chan M, Solomon K R, et al. Decay-Accelerating Factor (Cd55), a Glycosylphosphatidylinositol-Anchored Complement Regulatory Protein, Is a Receptor for Several Echoviruses. *Proceedings of the National Academy of Sciences of the United States of America*, 1994, 91(13): 6245-6248.

[47] Zhao X, Zhang G G, Liu S, et al. Human Neonatal Fc Receptor Is the Cellular Uncoating Receptor for Enterovirus B. *Cell*, 2019, 177(6): 1553-+.

[48] Morosky S, Wells A I, Lemon K, et al. The neonatal Fc receptor is a pan-echovirus receptor. *Proceedings of the National Academy of Sciences of the United States of America*, 2019, 116(9): 3758-3763.

[49] Wang K, Zheng B, Zhang L, et al. Serotype specific epitopes identified by neutralizing antibodies underpin immunogenic differences in Enterovirus B. *Nat Commun*, 2020, 11(1): 4419.

[50] Feng R, Wang L, Shi D, et al. Structural basis for neutralization of an anicteric hepatitis associated echovirus by a potent neutralizing antibody. *Cell Discov*, 2021, 7(1): 35.

[51] Qi S, Fu W, Fan J, et al. Structural Basis for the Immunogenicity of the C-Terminus of VP1 of Echovirus 3 Revealed by the Binding of a Neutralizing Antibody. *Viruses*, 2022, 14(11).

[52] Chen Z, Fischer E R, Kouiavskaia D, et al. Cross-neutralizing human anti-poliovirus antibodies bind the recognition site for cellular receptor. *Proc Natl Acad Sci USA*, 2013, 110(50): 20242-7.

[53] Strauss M, Schotte L, Thys B, et al. Five of Five VHHs Neutralizing Poliovirus Bind the Receptor-Binding Site. *J Virol*, 2016, 90(7): 3496-505.

[54] Liu Y, Sheng J, Baggen J, et al. Sialic acid-dependent cell entry of human enterovirus D68. *Nat Com*mun, 2015, 6: 8865.

[55] Baggen J, Thibaut H J, Staring J, et al. Enterovirus D68 receptor requirements unveiled by haploid genetics. *Proc Natl Acad Sci USA*, 2016, 113(5): 1399-404.

[56] Wei W, Guo H, Chang J, et al. ICAM-5/Telencephalin Is a Functional Entry Receptor for Enterovirus D68. *Cell Host Microbe*, 2016, 20(5): 631-641.

[57] Vogt M R, Fu J, Kose N, et al. Human antibodies neutralize enterovirus D68 and protect against infection and paralytic disease. *Sci Immunol*, 2020, 5(49).

[58] Zhang C, Xu C, Dai W, et al. Functional and structural characterization of a two-MAb cocktail for delayed treatment of enterovirus D68 infections. *Nat Commun*, 2021, 12(1): 2904.

[59] Plevka P, Lim P Y, Perera R, et al. Neutralizing antibodies can initiate genome release from human enterovirus 71. *Proceedings of the National Academy of Sciences of the United States of America*, 2014, 111(6): 2134-2139.

[60] Xu L, Zheng Q, Li S, et al. Atomic structures of Coxsackievirus A6 and its complex with a neutralizing antibody. *Nat Commun*, 2017, 8(1): 505.

[61] Lin J, Cheng N, Hogle J M, et al. Conformational shift of a major poliovirus antigen confirmed by immuno-cryogenic electron microscopy. *J Immunol*, 2013, 191(2): 884-91.

[62] Zheng Q, Zhu R, Xu L, et al. Atomic structures of enterovirus D68 in complex with two monoclonal antibodies define distinct mechanisms of viral neutralization. *Nat Microbiol*, 2019, 4(1): 124-133.

[63] Dong Y, Liu Y, Jiang W, et al. Antibody-induced uncoating of human rhinovirus B14. *Proc Natl Acad Sci USA*, 2017, 114(30): 8017-8022.

[64] Kim B, Eggel A, Tarchevskaya S S, et al. Accelerated disassembly of IgE-receptor complexes by a disruptive macromolecular inhibitor. *Nature*, 2012, 491(7425): 613-7.

[65] Eggel A, Baravalle G, Hobi G, et al. Accelerated dissociation of IgE-FcepsilonRI complexes by disruptive inhibitors actively desensitizes allergic effector cells. *J Allergy Clin Immunol*, 2014, 133(6): 1709-19 e8.

[66] Sim J, Sockolosky J T, Sangalang E, et al. Discovery of high affinity, pan-allelic, and pan-mammalian reactive antibodies against the myeloid checkpoint receptor SIRPalpha. *MAbs*, 2019, 11(6): 1036-1052.

[67] Huo J, Zhao Y, Ren J, et al. Neutralization of SARS-CoV-2 by Destruction of the Prefusion Spike. *Cell Host Microbe*, 2020, 28(3): 497.

[68] Lazear E, Whitbeck J C, Ponce-De-Leon M, et al. Antibody-induced conformational changes in herpes simplex virus glycoprotein gD reveal new targets for virus neutralization. *J Virol*, 2012, 86(3): 1563-76.

[69] Zheng Q, Jiang J, He M, et al. Viral neutralization by antibody-imposed physical disruption. *Proc Natl Acad Sci USA*, 2019, 116(52): 26933-26940.

[70] Xu L F, Zheng Q B, Zhu R, et al. Cryo-EM structures reveal the molecular basis of receptor-initiated coxsackievirus uncoating. *Cell Host & Microbe*, 2021, 29(3): 448-+.

[71] Wang X, Zhu L, Dang M, et al. Potent neutralization of hepatitis A virus reveals a receptor mimic mechanism and the receptor recognition site. *Proc Natl Acad Sci USA*, 2017, 114(4): 770-775.

[72] Wang X, Peng W, Ren J, et al. A sensor-adaptor mechanism for enterovirus uncoating from structures of EV71. *Nat Struct Mol Biol*, 2012, 19(4): 424-9.

[73] Ren J, Wang X, Hu Z, et al. Picornavirus uncoating intermediate captured in atomic detail. *Nat Commun*, 2013, 4: 1929.

[74] Pantaleo G, Correia B, Fenwick C, et al. Antibodies to combat viral infections: development strategies and progress. *Nat Rev Drug Discov*, 2022, 21(9): 676-696.

[75] Vogt M R, Dowd K A, Engle M, et al. Poorly neutralizing cross-reactive antibodies against the fusion loop of West Nile virus envelope protein protect in vivo via Fcgamma receptor and complement-dependent effector mechanisms. *J Virol*, 2011, 85(22): 11567-80.

[76] Kim A S, Kafai N M, Winkler E S, et al. Pan-protective anti-alphavirus human antibodies target a conserved E1 protein epitope. *Cell*, 2021, 184(17): 4414-4429 e19.

[77] Winkler E S, Gilchuk P, Yu J, et al. Human neutralizing antibodies against SARS-CoV-2 require intact Fc effector functions for optimal therapeutic protection. *Cell*, 2021, 184(7): 1804-1820 e16.

[78] Du R, An C, Yao X, et al. Non-neutralizing monoclonal antibody targeting VP2 EF loop of Coxsackievirus A16 can protect mice from lethal attack via Fc-dependent effector mechanism. *Emerg Microbes Infect,* 2023, 12(1): 2149352.

[79] Baum A, Ajithdoss D, Copin R, et al. REGN-COV2 antibodies prevent and treat SARS-CoV-2 infection in rhesus macaques and hamsters. *Science*, 2020, 370(6520): 1110-1115.

[80] Weinreich D M, Sivapalasingam S, Norton T, et al. REGN-COV2, a Neutralizing Antibody Cocktail, in Outpatients with Covid-19. *N Engl J Med*, 2021, 384(3): 238-251.

[81] Wec A Z, Bornholdt Z A, He S H, et al. Development of a Human Antibody Cocktail that Deploys Multiple Functions to Confer Pan-Ebolavirus Protection. *Cell Host & Microbe*, 2019, 25(1): 39-+.

[82] Takahashi S, Liao Q, Van Boeckel T P, et al. Hand, Foot, and Mouth Disease in China: Modeling Epidemic Dynamics of Enterovirus Serotypes and Implications for Vaccination. *PLoS Med,* 2016, 13(2): e1001958.

[83] Danthi P, Tosteson M, Li Q H, et al. Genome delivery and ion channel properties are altered in VP4 mutants of poliovirus. *J Virol*, 2003, 77(9): 5266-74.
[84] Panjwani A, Strauss M, Gold S, et al. Capsid protein VP4 of human rhinovirus induces membrane permeability by the formation of a size-selective multimeric pore. *PLoS Pathog*, 2014, 10(8): e1004294.
[85] Staring J, Von Castelmur E, Blomen V A, et al. PLA2G16 represents a switch between entry and clearance of Picornaviridae. *Nature*, 2017, 541(7637): 412-416.
[86] Liu Y, Sheng J, Fokine A, et al. Structure and inhibition of EV-D68, a virus that causes respiratory illness in children. *Science*, 2015, 347(6217): 71-4.
[87] Thibaut H J, De Palma A M, Neyts J. Combating enterovirus replication: state-of-the-art on antiviral research. *Biochem Pharmacol*, 2012, 83(2): 185-92.
[88] Xu J, Xu K, Jung S, et al. Nanobodies from camelid mice and llamas neutralize SARS-CoV-2 variants. *Nature*, 2021, 595(7866): 278-282.
[89] Xue X, Fan X, Qu Q, et al. Bioscreening and expression of a camel anti-CTGF VHH nanobody and its renaturation by a novel dialysis-dilution method. *AMB Express*, 2016, 6(1): 72.
[90] Ku Z, Shi J, Liu Q, et al. Development of murine monoclonal antibodies with potent neutralization effects on enterovirus 71. *J Virol Methods*, 2012, 186(1-2): 193-7.
[91] Ku Z, Ye X, Shi J, et al. Single Neutralizing Monoclonal Antibodies Targeting the VP1 GH Loop of Enterovirus 71 Inhibit both Virus Attachment and Internalization during Viral Entry. *J Virol*, 2015, 89(23): 12084-95.
[92] Ye X, Yang L, Jia J, et al. Development of sandwich ELISAs that can distinguish different types of coxsackievirus A16 viral particles. *Appl Microbiol Biotechnol*, 2016, 100(6): 2809-15.
[93] Chen Z, Chumakov K, Dragunsky E, et al. Chimpanzee-human monoclonal antibodies for treatment of chronic poliovirus excretors and emergency postexposure prophylaxis. *J Virol*, 2011, 85(9): 4354-62.

Chapter 4

Neutralizing Antibodies against Herpesvirus Entry Complex and Fusogen

Ling Zhong[1,2]
Wanlin Zhang[1,2]
Claude Krummenacher[3]
Qinjian Zhao[1]
and Xiao Zhang[1,*]

[1]College of Pharmacy, Chongqing Medical University, Chongqing, PR China
[2]State Key Laboratory of Oncology in South China,
Collaborative Innovation Center for Cancer Medicine,
Department of Experimental Research, Sun Yat-sen University Cancer Center,
Sun Yat-sen University, Guangzhou, Guangdong, PR China
[3]Department of Biological and Biomedical Sciences, Rowan University,
Glassboro, NJ, USA

Abstract

Herpesviruses lead to significant health challenges, notably through conditions like herpes, varicella, zoster, mononucleosis, and various cancers including Kaposi's sarcoma, nasopharyngeal carcinoma, and lymphoma. Yet, no approved treatments explicitly target the initial infections of herpesviruses. The herpesviruses' cell entry mechanism relies on the coordinated action of several glycoproteins and involves multiple host cell receptors. Glycoprotein B (gB) is essential for membrane fusion and gets activated by the entry complex, primarily formed of gH and gL. Given the central role of this entry complex and the fusogen in herpesvirus infections, antibodies neutralizing targeting

---

* Corresponding Author's Email: zhangxiao@cqmu.edu.cn.

In: Neutralizing Antibodies and their Role in Health and Disease
Editors: Chenguang Shen, Yang Yang and Minghui Yang
ISBN: 979-8-89113-541-3

the key epitopes on these glycoproteins offer a promising strategy to counteract herpesvirus infections.

Keywords: herpesvirus infection, gB, gH, gL, neutralizing antibodies

Introduction

Human herpesviruses are ubiquitous among human populations, which include three alpha-herpesviruses (herpes simplex viruses type 1 and 2 (HSV-1, HSV-2) and varicella-zoster virus (VZV)), four beta-herpesviruses (HHV-6A, HHV-6B, HHV-7 and human cytomegalovirus (HCMV)) and two gamma-herpesviruses (Kaposi's sarcoma-associated herpesviruses (KSHV) and Epstein-Barr virus (EBV)). Herpesviruses have evolved with their hosts over 60-80 million years and established life-long latency in host cells [1].

HSV primarily infects mucosa or skin epithelial cells and then establishes latency in sensory neurons. HSV can cause cold sores, genital herpes, stromal keratitis, eczema herpeticum, disseminated disease in the neonate, meningitis, and herpes simplex encephalitis [2]. VZV causes varicella (chickenpox) and then establishes latent infection in neurons. Reactivation of VZV causes zoster (shingles), which may lead to severe long-term postherpetic neuralgia [3]. Besides, HSV-1 and VZV reactivation may contribute to Alzheimer's disease [4]. HHV-6A and HHV-6B are also neurotropic and associated with multiple sclerosis and epilepsy, respectively [5]. Congenital HCMV infection causes sensorineural hearing loss and neurodevelopmental sequelae in infants [6]. HCMV disease is also a significant concern for solid organ transplant recipients and immunosuppressed individuals [7]. KSHV has a broad cell tropism linked to Kaposi's sarcoma (KS), primary effusion lymphoma, and multicentric Castleman disease [8]. EBV infects epithelial cells, B cells, NK/T cells, and macrophages. EBV, the first identified human oncogenic virus, is associated with many malignancies, including nasopharyngeal carcinoma, gastric carcinoma, Burkitt's lymphoma, and Hodgkin's lymphoma [9]. Besides, EBV infection most generally causes mononucleosis and has also recently been linked to multiple sclerosis [10-13]. EBV and HCMV reactivation have recently been reported to enhance COVID-19 severity [14-18]. Altogether, human herpesviruses cause heavy disease burdens. Nevertheless, no herpesviruses-specific vaccines or effective treatments that could block infection have been approved for clinical use except for vaccines against VZV.

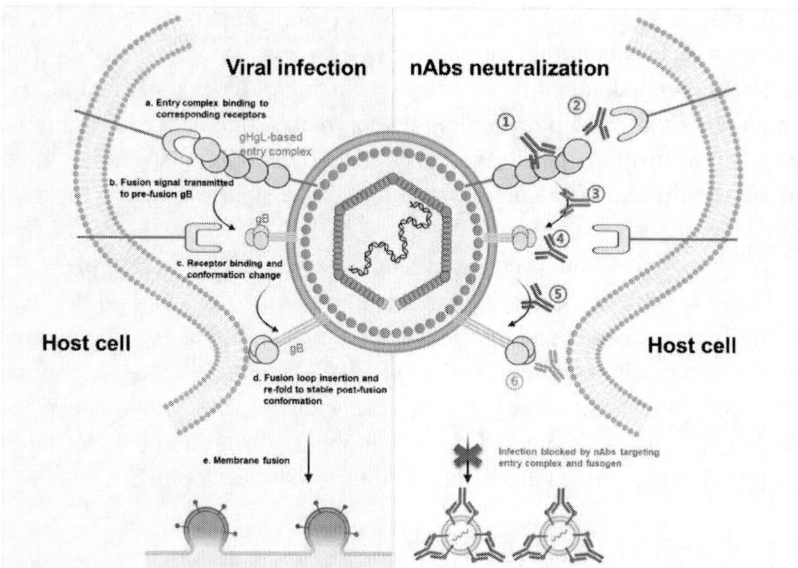

Figure 1. Key steps of the entry process of human herpesviruses and effects of nAbs targeting the entry complex and fusogen to block infection. Left: A generic herpesvirus key entry process is divided into 5 steps. a. A gHgL-based entry complex binds to specific cellular receptors. b. A fusion signal is transmitted from the entry complex to gB in its pre-fusion conformation. c. The pre-fusion gB binds to a putative receptor. d. gB inserts its hydrophobic fusion loops into a host cell membrane and re-folds into a stable post-fusion conformation. e. membrane fusion is completed and the capsid is released into the host cell. Right: multiple mechanisms used by nAbs targeting the entry complex and fusogen to block infection: (1) interference with the interactions within the entry complex preventing formation or leading to sdestabilization; (2) blocking of the interaction between the entry complex and cellular receptors; (3) inhibition of transmission of the fusion signal from the entry complex to the fusogen gB by preventing interactions between glycoproteins; (4) blocking of the interaction between gB and cellular receptors; (5) prevention of the conformation change of the fusogen gB; and (6) blocking the insertion of the fusion loop in the membrane of the target cell.

Unlike many other enveloped viruses, which use one or two glycoproteins to bind cellular receptors and accomplish membrane fusion, the process leading to fusion is more complicated in herpesviruses (Figure 1) [19, 20]. Human herpesviruses have evolved into a core entry machinery with two essential components to enter various cell types. One is the entry complex based on the gHgL heterodimer and the other is the fusogen gB, which actively promotes membrane fusion. During herpesvirus infection, the virus first attaches non-specifically to molecules at the surface of cells, usually glycosaminoglycans, and then binds to specific host cell receptors to lessen the distance between the virus and target cells and activate its fusion machinery. Second, an entry complex consisting of at least gH and gL, often containing specific receptor-binding glycoproteins, interacts with receptors to change conformation. Third, the entry gB activates the fusogen complex to undergo conformation changes from pre- to post-fusion states to achieve membrane fusion.

To summarize, entry complex and fusogen play crucial roles in the herpesvirus entry process [21]. Hence, neutralizing antibodies (nAbs) targeting entry complex and fusogen are potential prophylactic and therapeutic reagents, especially considering the lack of effective treatments for many human herpesviruses. Moreover, the characterization of nAbs can provide valuable information about functional epitope footprints and the mechanisms of neutralization, which will further guide vaccine development.

Neutralizing Antibodies Targeting Entry Complex

The entry complex of different herpesvirus is distinct and contains several other non-conserved proteins except for heterodimer gHgL. gD is the specific and essential receptor-binding glycoprotein functionally associated with gHgL during HSV infection. At the same time, the gHgL complex of VZV is sufficient to initiate the entry process and then trigger gB [22, 23]. gO or three smaller UL proteins (UL128, UL130 and UL131A) binding to gHgL to form a trimeric gHgL/gO complex or a pentameric gHgL/UL128/UL130/UL131A complex is essential for HCMV infection and tetrameric gHgL/gQ1/gQ2 is entry complex for HHV-6A and 6B [24, 25]. EBV carries a gHgL/gp42 complex or a gHgL complex responsible for B cell or epithelial cell entry [26]. Many nAbs against the entry complex of herpesvirus have been characterized.

Neutralizing Antibodies Targeting Alpha-Herpesvirus Entry Complex

In the case of the HSV entry complex, nAbs could be divided into four clusters according to their neutralizing mechanisms. Cluster 1 nAbs neutralize HSV infection through interfering interactions between gD and its receptors. gD-specific nAbs 1D3, CH42, and CH43 inhibit the interaction between gD and herpesvirus entry mediator (HVEM), while 4A3, LP2, and MC23 block gD-nectin interaction [27-29]. DL11 and E317 block HSV infection by inhibiting gD-HVEM and gD-nectin interactions [27, 30]. Cluster 2 nAbs block the interaction between gD and gHgL, which contains gD-specific nAb MC5 and gH-specific nAbs CHL17, CHL27 and CHL32 [27, 31]. Cluster 3 nAbs interfere with the interaction between gHgL and gB, such as LP11 targeting gH domain H1/2 [32]. Cluster 4 nAbs, including gH-specific nAb CHL21 and gD-specific nAbs m27f and MC2, affect the post-entry step [27, 31, 33]. M Mice treated with 3 mg/kg or higher concentrations of m27f were wholly protected from lethal HSV-2 infection [33]. Besides, 100% of the mice injected intraperitoneally with 30-450 μg of CH42/CH43 survived after a deadly challenge with HSV-1 inoculated by corneal scarification [28]. Furthermore, gD-specific nAb HSV8 is being tested in clinical trials to reduce the vaginal transmission of HSV (NCT02579083). Another gD-specific nAb E317 (UB-621) is being evaluated in clinical trials for reducing the HSV-2 genital shedding rate and reducing adult recurrent HSV-2 infections of the genitals (NCT02346760, NCT03595995, NCT04714060 and NCT04979975).

As for VZV, the nAbs targeting VZV gH or gHgL are identified as mAb206 (domain H1A), IgG-24 (domain H1/2) and IgG-RC, IgG-94 (domain H1 and gL) [23]. BALB/c mice immunized with gHgL/Fab-RC complex showed a significant reduction of neutralizing antibody levels compared with mice immunized with gHgL, suggesting the Fab-RC domain masked important neutralizing epitopes on gHgL [23].

Neutralizing Antibodies Targeting Beta-Herpesvirus Entry Complex

A large number of nAbs targeting the HCMV entry complexes have been characterized. HCMV pentameric complex (PC; gHgL/UL128/UL130/UL131A) contains four immunogenic regions (IR) and eight immunogenic sites [34, 35]. IR1, including four immunogenic sites, consists of UL128, UL130, and UL131A. IR2 contains gL and N terminals of gH, and immunogenic sites 5 and 6 are located in this region. IR3 includes one immunogenic site composed of the C terminal of gH, while IR4 contains a linear immunogenic site located at the first 40 amino acids of gH. IR1-specific nAbs showed the most potent neutralizing ability in HCMV infection of epithelial cells instead of fibroblast cells, while IR4-specific nAbs only inhibited HCMV infection of epithelial cells [35]. Most IR2- and IR3- specific nAbs showed similar neutralizing ability of HCMV infection of epithelial cells and fibroblast cells, indicating the typical roles of IR2 and IR3 in the HCMV infection process [35]. nAbs targeting gHgL showed similar binding ability to PC and gHgLgO trimer, which confirmed these epitopes are conserved in the two kinds of entry complex [36]. Although sera of patients infected with HCMV contain trimer- and pentamer-specific antibodies, no nAbs binding to gO have been reported due to its extensive glycosylation and less conservative [37]. Neutralizing mechanisms of nAbs targeting HCMV entry complex contain block the interactions between PC and receptors (1-103, 2C12, 7I13, 9I6, 10P3 and 15D8), interfering interactions between gHgL and gB (4N10, 8I21, 3G16 and 13H11) and perturbing PC dimerization (1-32, 2-18 and 2-25) or gHgL dimerization (MSL-109) [34, 36, 38-41]. MSL-109 targeting gH domain II/III is being tested in clinical trials [42-44]. Although MSL-109 failed to reduce HCMV infection in allogeneic hematopoietic stem cell transplantation recipients, the combination of MSL-109 and MCMV3068A reduced HCMV infection and HCMV-associated diseases in the kidney transplant recipients [43, 44].

Although there is currently no established prevention or treatment for HHV-6, it has been previously demonstrated that a mouse mAb against gQ1-residue 484 to 496 (KH-1), and a mouse-derived mAb against gH-domain II (OHV-3) have strong neutralizing activity against HHV-6B infection [45, 46]. Furthermore, nAbs gH1-1, AgL3 and gQ2-4 block both the HHV-6A and HHV-6B infection [45].

Neutralizing Antibodies Targeting Gamma-Herpesvirus Entry Complex

Neutralizing Abs that target the EBV entry complexes include epithelial cell-specific nAbs against gH-domain II (CL40), gH-domain IV (CL59) and gL (E1D1), B cell-specific nAbs target gp42 (F-2-1, G-3-1) and dual-specific nAbs have been found against gH-domain I/II (AMMO1, 769B10, 1D8), and gH-domain IV (6H2) [47-52]. Administration of CL40, CL59, AMMO1, 1D8, 769B10 and 6H2 protected humanized mice from lethal EBV challenge [51-54]. Thus, these nAbs are potential prophylactic agents to prevent EBV infection in human.

Neutralizing Antibodies against Fusogen gB

The conserved fusogen is natively a homotrimer with two conformation structures, pre-fusion and post-fusion. GB consists of a single-pass transmembrane domain, a membrane-proximal region, and a large ectodomain subdivided into 5 structural domains. The immunogenicity of each domain is distinct. Domain I, with the pleckstrin-like region, is located at the base of the molecule. It displays extended β-sheets and contains two hydrophobic fusion loops responsible for insertion into the cell membrane [55-58]. Domain II also adopts a pleckstrin-like structure, which may be the binding site for host cell membrane phospholipids [59, 60]. Domain III forms a long helical domain involving a coiled-coil structure at the center of the gB trimer. The flexible domain IV forms a crown at the top of post-fusion gB and Domain V is extended from the top to the bottom of post-fusion gB. Co-receptors for gB have been reported, including neuropilin 1 [61], paired immunoglobulin-like type 2 receptor-α [62, 63], non-muscle myosin heavy chain IIA [64] and myelin-associated glycoprotein [65].

nAbs targeting gB are potential prophylactic and therapeutic reagents since gB is the fusogen for herpesvirus infection of all susceptible cell types. Characterization of neutralizing antibodies against gB can provide valuable information about functional epitope footprints, which will further guide vaccine development.

Neutralizing Antibodies against HSV and VZV gB

HSV-1 gB contains four functional regions (FRs) determined by monoclonal antibodies (mAbs) [66]. FR1 includes domain I and residues 697-725 in domain V and is detected by mAbs SS55, SS56, SS118, SS106 and SS144. Antibodies targeting FR1 permanently neutralize but do not directly bind to fusion loops [67]. Besides, nAb 2C against domain I inhibit HSV infection by cross-linking HSV gB [68]. Two clinical trials about the humanized nAb, hu2C are being launched to determine the protection efficiency of orolabial lesions and anogenital lesions (NCT04539483; NCT04165122). FR2 includes three overlapping epitopes from domain II, and antibodies such as H1838, H1781, and C226 bind to this region [66]. FR3 contains residues from domain IV near domain III and antibodies such as SS10, SS67, SS68 and SS69 target this region [66]. The N-terminal FR4 is formed by residues 31-43 and is recognized by antibody H1817 [66].

Only one nAb targeting VZV gB is reported. The human monoclonal antibody 93K targeting VZV gB domain IV efficiently blocks VZV infection and membrane fusion *in vitro* [69].

Neutralizing Antibodies against HCMV gB

HCMV gB contains five antigenic domains (AD) defined by mAbs. AD-1 is located within domain IV (residues 552 to 635) and is highly immunogenic because most residues are exposed, but antibodies to AD-1 are not all neutralizing [70-72]. The epitopes of nAbs may be exposed on the pre-fusion structure, and those of non-neutralizing antibodies may be specific for the post-fusion conformation. AD-2 contains two regions, including residues 68-77, recognized by nAbs, and residues 50-54, which elicit non-neutralizing antibodies [73, 74]. Two AD-2-specific TCN-202 and TRL345 clinical trials have been launched (NCT01594437; NCT05408091). Besides, a few individuals elicited AD-2-specific nAbs after natural infection, and the neutralizing ability usually relies on bivalency for neutralization [74, 75]. To date, no reported nAbs target the AD-3 region that contains linear epitopes of TMD and cytoplasmic tail [76]. AD-4, located at domain II (residues 121-132 and 44-438), and AD-5, located within domain I, are recognized by many nAbs [76]. These include SM1-6, SM3-1, SM4-5, SM5-1, SM6-5, SM11-17 and SM5-1 binding to AD-4 and SM10, 1G2 and SM12 targeting AD-5 [76-79]. Besides, AD-4 and AD-5 are targeted by more than 90% and 50% of sera from HCMV carriers, respectively [76]. Thus, AD-4 and AD-5 are promising antigens for HCMV vaccine development. Furthermore, AD-4 and AD-5 maintained similar structures in pre- and post-fusion structure of gB [80]. Part of AD-1 is buried in the pre-fusion structure, while the structure of AD-2 remains unsolved in both the pre-and post-fusion structure [80].

Neutralizing Antibodies against EBV gB

In contrast to the plethora of characterized antibodies against HSV and HCMV, only a handful of mAbs have been reported for EBV gB. These include neutralizing antibodies AMMO5, 8A9, 8C12, 3A3 targeting domain II, neutralizing antibody 3A5 targeting domain IV and non-neutralizing antibodies AMMO2, AMMO3, AMMO4 and CL55 [50, 81-83]. 3A3 and 3A5 completely neutralized EBV infection in the humanized mouse model [83]. 3A3 inhibits EBV infection by interfering with the interaction between gB and receptor neuropilin 1, while 3A5 neutralizes EBV infection by hindering gB activation [83]. Importantly, the epitopes recognized by 3A3 and 3A5 are immunodominant in naturally infected individuals [83].

Discussion

Screening of neutralizing anti-glycoprotein antibodies will yield important data to guide vaccine development and immunoglobulin-based therapies. Antibodies targeting the human herpesvirus entry complex and fusogen neutralize herpesvirus infection through different mechanisms (Figure 1). nAbs found protective in vivo in animal models are worthy of further evaluation in clinical trials alone and in combinations.

Up to now, all the reported neutralizing or non-neutralizing antibodies target post-fusion gB. Immunization with pre-fusion gB is anticipated to elicit more effective neutralizing antibodies, but the production of stable pre-fusion gB proteins must be improved. Except for HSV-1 and HCMV, the native pre-fusion gB structures remain unknown, and the mass expression of pre-fusion gB is still limited [80, 84]. Therefore, scientific and technological advances are needed to use pre-fusion gB as an antigen for specific antibody screening. Another required advance relates to our understanding of the transmission of the fusion signal from receptor binding of entry complex to effective membrane fusion. Although the neutralizing mechanism of several nAbs is thought to block entry complex-fusogen interactions, the detailed interaction sites and structure of the entry complex-fusogen remain unknown.

Since herpesvirus infection involves multiple envelop glycoproteins, multi-specific antibodies or antibody cocktails are more promising strategies for completely preventing infection or efficiently treating herpesvirus-associated diseases. A bispecific antibody targeting HCMV gB and gHgL/UL128/UL130/UL131A showed improved neutralization breadth and potency [85]. Besides, a bispecific T cell engager antibody, through the combination of anti-CD3 and anti-gB antibody, efficiently eradicate the HCMV-infected cells [86, 87]. As for the cocktail treatment, nAbs targeting epitopes far from each other have synergistic neutralizing effects and, therefore, provide potential therapeutic options as cocktails [88]. However, the optimum selection of nAbs for cocktail treatment remains to be determined. A combination of gB-specific LJ538 and PC-specific LPJ539 antibodies failed to prevent HCMV reactivation in allogeneic hematopoietic stem cell transplant recipients [89].

In conclusion, while there are still questions surrounding the neutralizing functions of certain nAbs and the neutralizing epitopes of pre-fusion gB, analyzing and understanding nAbs in human herpesvirus offers valuable insights for the logical creation of vaccines and inhibitors. nAbs also hold the potential as critical components in immunoglobulin-driven treatments or preventive methods. Future studies on herpesvirus-specific nAbs should also explore strategies like bispecific or multi-specific antibodies and combinations.

References

[1] Davison, A. J., Dargan, D. J., Stow, N. D., Fundamental and accessory systems in herpesviruses. *Antiviral Res* 2002, 56, (1), 1-11.

[2] Zhu, S., Viejo-Borbolla, A., Pathogenesis and virulence of herpes simplex virus. *Virulence* 2021, 12, (1), 2670-2702.

[3] Gershon, A. A., Breuer, J., Cohen, J. I., Cohrs, R. J., Gershon, M. D., Gilden, D., Grose, C., Hambleton, S., Kennedy, P. G., Oxman, M. N., Seward, J. F., Yamanishi, K., Varicella zoster virus infection. *Nat Rev Dis Primers* 2015, 1, 15016.

[4] Cairns, D. M., Itzhaki, R. F., Kaplan, D. L., Potential Involvement of Varicella Zoster Virus in Alzheimer's Disease via Reactivation of Quiescent Herpes Simplex Virus Type 1. *J Alzheimers Dis* 2022.

[5] Dunn, N., Kharlamova, N., Fogdell-Hahn, A., The role of herpesvirus 6A and 6B in multiple sclerosis and epilepsy. *Scand J Immunol* 2020, 92, (6), e12984.

[6] Boppana, S. B., Ross, S. A., Fowler, K. B., Congenital cytomegalovirus infection: clinical outcome. *Clin Infect Dis* 2013, 57 Suppl 4, S178-81.

[7] Fulkerson, H. L., Nogalski, M. T., Collins-McMillen, D., Yurochko, A. D., Overview of Human Cytomegalovirus Pathogenesis. *Methods Mol Biol* 2021, 2244, 1-18.

[8] Wen, K. W., Damania, B., Kaposi sarcoma-associated herpesvirus (KSHV): molecular biology and oncogenesis. *Cancer Lett* 2010, 289, (2), 140-50.

[9] Khan, G., Fitzmaurice, C., Naghavi, M., Ahmed, L. A., Global and regional incidence, mortality and disability-adjusted life-years for Epstein-Barr virus-attributable malignancies, 1990-2017. *BMJ Open* 2020, 10, (8), e037505.

[10] Bjornevik, K., Cortese, M., Healy, B. C., Kuhle, J., Mina, M. J., Leng, Y., Elledge, S. J., Niebuhr, D. W., Scher, A. I., Munger, K. L., Ascherio, A., Longitudinal analysis reveals high prevalence of Epstein-Barr virus associated with multiple sclerosis. *Science* 2022, 375, (6578), 296-301.

[11] Lanz, T. V., Brewer, R. C., Ho, P. P., Moon, J. S., Jude, K. M., Fernandez, D., Fernandes, R. A., Gomez, A. M., Nadj, G. S., Bartley, C. M., Schubert, R. D., Hawes, I. A., Vazquez, S. E., Iyer, M., Zuchero, J. B., Teegen, B., Dunn, J. E., Lock, C. B., Kipp, L. B., Cotham, V. C., Ueberheide, B. M., Aftab, B. T., Anderson, M. S., DeRisi, J. L., Wilson, M. R., Bashford-Rogers, R. J. M., Platten, M., Garcia, K. C., Steinman, L., Robinson, W. H., Clonally expanded B cells in multiple sclerosis bind EBV EBNA1 and GlialCAM. *Nature* 2022, 603, (7900), 321-327.

[12] Luzuriaga, K., Sullivan, J. L., Infectious mononucleosis. *N Engl J Med* 2010, 362, (21), 1993-2000.

[13] Zhong, L., Zhao, Q., Zhang, X., Unmasking the Enigma: Epstein-Barr Virus as a Primary Trigger in Multiple Sclerosis. *J Autoimmune Disord* 2023, 9, (2), 31.

[14] Paolucci, S., Cassaniti, I., Novazzi, F., Fiorina, L., Piralla, A., Comolli, G., Bruno, R., Maserati, R., Gulminetti, R., Novati, S., Mojoli, F., Baldanti, F., San Matteo Pavia, C.-T. F., EBV DNA increase in COVID-19 patients with impaired lymphocyte subpopulation count. *Int J Infect Dis* 2021, 104, 315-319.

[15] Chen, T., Song, J., Liu, H., Zheng, H., Chen, C., Positive Epstein-Barr virus detection in coronavirus disease 2019 (COVID-19) patients. *Sci Rep* 2021, 11, (1), 10902.

[16] Nadeem, A., Suresh, K., Awais, H., Waseem, S., Epstein-Barr Virus Coinfection in COVID-19. *J Investig Med High Impact Case Rep* 2021, 9, 23247096211040626.

[17] Soderberg-Naucler, C., Does reactivation of cytomegalovirus contribute to severe COVID-19 disease? *Immun Ageing* 2021, 18, (1), 12.

[18] Gold, J. E., Okyay, R. A., Licht, W. E., Hurley, D. J., Investigation of Long COVID Prevalence and Its Relationship to Epstein-Barr Virus Reactivation. *Pathogens* 2021, 10, (6).

[19] Harrison, S. C., Viral membrane fusion. *Virology* 2015, 479-480, 498-507.

[20] Eisenberg, R. J., Atanasiu, D., Cairns, T. M., Gallagher, J. R., Krummenacher, C., Cohen, G. H., Herpes virus fusion and entry: a story with many characters. *Viruses* 2012, 4, (5), 800-32.

[21] Zhong, L., Zhang, W., Krummenacher, C., Chen, Y., Zheng, Q., Zhao, Q., Zeng, M. S., Xia, N., Zeng, Y. X., Xu, M., Zhang, X., Targeting herpesvirus entry complex and fusogen glycoproteins with prophylactic and therapeutic agents. *Trends Microbiol* 2023, 31, (8), 788-804.

[22] Fan, Q., Kopp, S., Connolly, S. A., Muller, W. J., Longnecker, R., Mapping sites of herpes simplex virus type 1 glycoprotein D that permit insertions and impact gD and gB receptors usage. *Sci Rep* 2017, 7, 43712.

[23] Xing, Y., Oliver, S. L., Nguyen, T., Ciferri, C., Nandi, A., Hickman, J., Giovani, C., Yang, E., Palladino, G., Grose, C., Uematsu, Y., Lilja, A. E., Arvin, A. M., Carfi, A., A site of varicella-zoster virus vulnerability identified by structural studies of neutralizing antibodies bound to the glycoprotein complex gHgL. *Proc Natl Acad Sci USA* 2015, 112, (19), 6056-61.

[24] Akkapaiboon, P., Mori, Y., Sadaoka, T., Yonemoto, S., Yamanishi, K., Intracellular Processing of Human Herpesvirus 6 Glycoproteins Q1 and Q2 into Tetrameric Complexes Expressed on the Viral Envelope. *Journal of Virology* 2004, 78, (15), 7969-7983.

[25] Zhou, M., Lanchy, J. M., Ryckman, B. J., Human Cytomegalovirus gH/gL/gO Promotes the Fusion Step of Entry into All Cell Types, whereas gH/gL/UL128-131 Broadens Virus Tropism through a Distinct Mechanism. *J Virol* 2015, 89, (17), 8999-9009.

[26] Li, Q., Turk, S. M., Hutt-Fletcher, L. M., The Epstein-Barr virus (EBV) BZLF2 gene product associates with the gH and gL homologs of EBV and carries an epitope critical to infection of B cells but not of epithelial cells. *J Virol* 1995, 69, (7), 3987-94.

[27] Cairns, T. M., Ditto, N. T., Atanasiu, D., Lou, H., Brooks, B. D., Saw, W. T., Eisenberg, R. J., Cohen, G. H., Surface Plasmon Resonance Reveals Direct Binding of Herpes Simplex Virus Glycoproteins gH/gL to gD and Locates a gH/gL Binding Site on gD. *J Virol* 2019, 93, (15).

[28] Wang, K., Tomaras, G. D., Jegaskanda, S., Moody, M. A., Liao, H. X., Goodman, K. N., Berman, P. W., Rerks-Ngarm, S., Pitisuttithum, P., Nitayapan, S., Kaewkungwal, J., Haynes, B. F., Cohen, J. I., Monoclonal Antibodies, Derived from Humans Vaccinated with the RV144 HIV Vaccine Containing the HVEM Binding Domain of Herpes Simplex Virus (HSV) Glycoprotein D, Neutralize HSV Infection, Mediate Antibody-Dependent Cellular Cytotoxicity, and Protect Mice from Ocular Challenge with HSV-1. *J Virol* 2017, 91, (19).

[29] Tian, R., Ju, F., Yu, M., Liang, Z., Xu, Z., Zhao, M., Qin, Y., Lin, Y., Huang, X., Chang, Y., Li, S., Ren, W., Lin, C., Xia, N., Huang, C., A potent neutralizing and protective antibody against a conserved continuous epitope on HSV glycoprotein D. *Antiviral Res* 2022, 201, 105298.

[30] Lee, C. C., Lin, L. L., Chan, W. E., Ko, T. P., Lai, J. S., Wang, A. H., Structural basis for the antibody neutralization of herpes simplex virus. *Acta Crystallogr D Biol Crystallogr* 2013, 69, (Pt 10), 1935-45.

[31] Cairns, T. M., Atanasiu, D., Saw, W. T., Lou, H., Whitbeck, J. C., Ditto, N. T., Bruun, B., Browne, H., Bennett, L., Wu, C., Krummenacher, C., Brooks, B. D., Eisenberg, R. J., Cohen, G. H., Localization of the Interaction Site of Herpes Simplex Virus Glycoprotein D (gD) on the Membrane Fusion Regulator, gH/gL. *J Virol* 2020, 94, (20).

[32] Chowdary, T. K., Cairns, T. M., Atanasiu, D., Cohen, G. H., Eisenberg, R. J., Heldwein, E. E., Crystal structure of the conserved herpesvirus fusion regulator complex gH-gL. *Nat Struct Mol Biol* 2010, 17, (7), 882-8.

[33] Du, R., Wang, L., Xu, H., Wang, Z., Zhang, T., Wang, M., Ning, Y., Deng, F., Hu, Z., Wang, H., Li, Y., A novel glycoprotein D-specific monoclonal antibody neutralizes herpes simplex virus. *Antiviral Res* 2017, 147, 131-141.

[34] Kschonsak, M., Johnson, M. C., Schelling, R., Green, E. M., Rougé, L., Ho, H., Patel, N., Kilic, C., Kraft, E., Arthur, C. P., Rohou, A. L., Comps-Agrar, L., Martinez-Martin, N., Perez, L., Payandeh, J., Ciferri, C., Structural basis for HCMV Pentamer receptor recognition and antibody neutralization. *Sci Adv* 2022, 8, (10), eabm2536.

[35] Ha, S., Li, F., Troutman, M. C., Freed, D. C., Tang, A., Loughney, J. W., Wang, D., Wang, I. M., Vlasak, J., Nickle, D. C., Rustandi, R. R., Hamm, M., DePhillips, P. A., Zhang, N., McLellan, J. S., Zhu, H., Adler, S. P., McVoy, M. A., An, Z., Fu, T.

M., Neutralization of Diverse Human Cytomegalovirus Strains Conferred by Antibodies Targeting Viral gH/gL/pUL128-131 Pentameric Complex. *J Virol* 2017, 91, (7).

[36] Ciferri, C., Chandramouli, S., Leitner, A., Donnarumma, D., Cianfrocco, M. A., Gerrein, R., Friedrich, K., Aggarwal, Y., Palladino, G., Aebersold, R., Norais, N., Settembre, E. C., Carfi, A., Antigenic Characterization of the HCMV gH/gL/gO and Pentamer Cell Entry Complexes Reveals Binding Sites for Potently Neutralizing Human Antibodies. *PLoS Pathog* 2015, 11, (10), e1005230.

[37] Vanarsdall, A. L., Chin, A. L., Liu, J., Jardetzky, T. S., Mudd, J. O., Orloff, S. L., Streblow, D., Mussi-Pinhata, M. M., Yamamoto, A. Y., Duarte, G., Britt, W. J., Johnson, D. C., HCMV trimer- and pentamer-specific antibodies synergize for virus neutralization but do not correlate with congenital transmission. *Proc Natl Acad Sci USA* 2019, 116, (9), 3728-3733.

[38] Fouts, A. E., Comps-Agrar, L., Stengel, K. F., Ellerman, D., Schoeffler, A. J., Warming, S., Eaton, D. L., Feierbach, B., Mechanism for neutralizing activity by the anti-CMV gH/gL monoclonal antibody MSL-109. *Proc Natl Acad Sci USA* 2014, 111, (22), 8209-14.

[39] Chandramouli, S., Malito, E., Nguyen, T., Luisi, K., Donnarumma, D., Xing, Y., Norais, N., Yu, D., Carfi, A., Structural basis for potent antibody-mediated neutralization of human cytomegalovirus. *Science immunology* 2017, 2, (12).

[40] Ciferri, C., Chandramouli, S., Donnarumma, D., Nikitin, P. A., Cianfrocco, M. A., Gerrein, R., Feire, A. L., Barnett, S. W., Lilja, A. E., Rappuoli, R., Norais, N., Settembre, E. C., Carfi, A., Structural and biochemical studies of HCMV gH/gL/gO and Pentamer reveal mutually exclusive cell entry complexes. *Proc Natl Acad Sci USA* 2015, 112, (6), 1767-72.

[41] Wrapp, D., Ye, X., Ku, Z., Su, H., Jones, H. G., Wang, N., Mishra, A. K., Freed, D. C., Li, F., Tang, A., Li, L., Jaijyan, D. K., Zhu, H., Wang, D., Fu, T. M., Zhang, N., An, Z., McLellan, J. S., Structural basis for HCMV Pentamer recognition by neuropilin 2 and neutralizing antibodies. *Sci Adv* 2022, 8, (10), eabm2546.

[42] Borucki, M. J., Spritzler, J., Asmuth, D. M., Gnann, J., Hirsch, M. S., Nokta, M., Aweeka, F., Nadler, P. I., Sattler, F., Alston, B., Nevin, T. T., Owens, S., Waterman, K., Hubbard, L., Caliendo, A., Pollard, R. B., Team, A., A phase II, double-masked, randomized, placebo-controlled evaluation of a human monoclonal anti-Cytomegalovirus antibody (MSL-109) in combination with standard therapy versus standard therapy alone in the treatment of AIDS patients with Cytomegalovirus retinitis. *Antiviral Res* 2004, 64, (2), 103-11.

[43] Ishida, J. H., Patel, A., Mehta, A. K., Gatault, P., McBride, J. M., Burgess, T., Derby, M. A., Snydman, D. R., Emu, B., Feierbach, B., Fouts, A. E., Maia, M., Deng, R., Rosenberger, C. M., Gennaro, L. A., Striano, N. S., Liao, X. C., Tavel, J. A., Phase 2 Randomized, Double-Blind, Placebo-Controlled Trial of RG7667, a Combination Monoclonal Antibody, for Prevention of Cytomegalovirus Infection in High-Risk Kidney Transplant Recipients. *Antimicrob Agents Chemother* 2017, 61, (2).

[44] Boeckh, M., Bowden, R. A., Storer, B., Chao, N. J., Spielberger, R., Tierney, D. K., Gallez-Hawkins, G., Cunningham, T., Blume, K. G., Levitt, D., Zaia, J. A., Randomized, placebo-controlled, double-blind study of a cytomegalovirus-specific

monoclonal antibody (MSL-109) for prevention of cytomegalovirus infection after allogeneic hematopoietic stem cell transplantation. *Biol Blood Marrow Transplant* 2001, 7, (6), 343-51.

[45] Kawabata, A., Oyaizu, H., Maeki, T., Tang, H., Yamanishi, K., Mori, Y., Analysis of a neutralizing antibody for human herpesvirus 6B reveals a role for glycoprotein Q1 in viral entry. *J Virol* 2011, 85, (24), 12962-71.

[46] Wang, B., Nishimura, M., Maekawa, Y., Kotari, T., Okuno, T., Mori, Y., Humanization of Murine Neutralizing Antibodies against Human Herpesvirus 6B. *J Virol* 2019, 93, (10).

[47] Sathiyamoorthy, K., Hu, Y. X., Mohl, B. S., Chen, J., Longnecker, R., Jardetzky, T. S., Structural basis for Epstein-Barr virus host cell tropism mediated by gp42 and gHgL entry glycoproteins. *Nat Commun* 2016, 7, 13557.

[48] Sathiyamoorthy, K., Jiang, J., Mohl, B. S., Chen, J., Zhou, Z. H., Longnecker, R., Jardetzky, T. S., Inhibition of EBV-mediated membrane fusion by anti-gHgL antibodies. *Proc Natl Acad Sci USA* 2017, 114, (41), E8703-E8710.

[49] Strnad, B. C., Schuster, T., Klein, R., Hopkins, R. F., 3rd, Witmer, T., Neubauer, R. H., Rabin, H., Production and characterization of monoclonal antibodies against the Epstein-Barr virus membrane antigen. *J Virol* 1982, 41, (1), 258-64.

[50] Snijder, J., Ortego, M. S., Weidle, C., Stuart, A. B., Gray, M. D., McElrath, M. J., Pancera, M., Veesler, D., McGuire, A. T., An Antibody Targeting the Fusion Machinery Neutralizes Dual-Tropic Infection and Defines a Site of Vulnerability on Epstein-Barr Virus. *Immunity* 2018, 48, (4), 799-811 e9.

[51] Zhu, Q. Y., Shan, S., Yu, J., Peng, S. Y., Sun, C., Zuo, Y., Zhong, L. Y., Yan, S. M., Zhang, X., Yang, Z., Peng, Y. J., Shi, X., Cao, S. M., Wang, X., Zeng, M. S., Zhang, L., A potent and protective human neutralizing antibody targeting a novel vulnerable site of Epstein-Barr virus. *Nat Commun* 2021, 12, (1), 6624.

[52] Hong, J., Zhong, L., Zheng, Q., Wu, Q., Zha, Z., Wei, D., Chen, H., Zhang, W., Zhang, S., Huang, Y., Chen, K., Chen, J., Li, S., Zeng, M. S., Zeng, Y. X., Xia, N., Zhang, X., Xu, M., Chen, Y., A Neutralizing Antibody Targeting gH Provides Potent Protection against EBV Challenge In Vivo. *J Virol* 2022, 96, (8), e0007522.

[53] Singh, S., Homad, L. J., Akins, N. R., Stoffers, C. M., Lackhar, S., Malhi, H., Wan, Y. H., Rawlings, D. J., McGuire, A. T., Neutralizing Antibodies Protect against Oral Transmission of Lymphocryptovirus. *Cell Rep Med* 2020, 1, (3).

[54] Chen, W. H., Kim, J., Bu, W., Board, N. L., Tsybovsky, Y., Wang, Y., Hostal, A., Andrews, S. F., Gillespie, R. A., Choe, M., Stephens, T., Yang, E. S., Pegu, A., Peterson, C. E., Fisher, B. E., Mascola, J. R., Pittaluga, S., McDermott, A. B., Kanekiyo, M., Joyce, M. G., Cohen, J. I., Epstein-Barr virus gH/gL has multiple sites of vulnerability for virus neutralization and fusion inhibition. *Immunity* 2022, 55, (11), 2135-2148 e6.

[55] Falanga, A., Tarallo, R., Vitiello, G., Vitiello, M., Perillo, E., Cantisani, M., D'Errico, G., Galdiero, M., Galdiero, S., Biophysical characterization and membrane interaction of the two fusion loops of glycoprotein B from herpes simplex type I virus. *PLoS One* 2012, 7, (2), e32186.

[56] Heldwein, E. E., Lou, H., Bender, F. C., Cohen, G. H., Eisenberg, R. J., Harrison, S. C., Crystal structure of glycoprotein B from herpes simplex virus 1. *Science* 2006, 313, (5784), 217-20.

[57] Sharma, S., Wisner, T. W., Johnson, D. C., Heldwein, E. E., HCMV gB shares structural and functional properties with gB proteins from other herpesviruses. *Virology* 2013, 435, (2), 239-49.

[58] Backovic, M., Longnecker, R., Jardetzky, T. S., Structure of a trimeric variant of the Epstein-Barr virus glycoprotein B. *Proc Natl Acad Sci USA* 2009, 106, (8), 2880-5.

[59] Lemmon, M. A., Pleckstrin homology domains: not just for phosphoinositides. *Biochem Soc Trans* 2004, 32, (Pt 5), 707-11.

[60] Lemmon, M. A., Membrane recognition by phospholipid-binding domains. *Nat Rev Mol Cell Biol* 2008, 9, (2), 99-111.

[61] Wang, H. B., Zhang, H., Zhang, J. P., Li, Y., Zhao, B., Feng, G. K., Du, Y., Xiong, D., Zhong, Q., Liu, W. L., Du, H., Li, M. Z., Huang, W. L., Tsao, S. W., Hutt-Fletcher, L., Zeng, Y. X., Kieff, E., Zeng, M. S., Neuropilin 1 is an entry factor that promotes EBV infection of nasopharyngeal epithelial cells. *Nat Commun* 2015, 6, 6240.

[62] Satoh, T., Arii, J., Suenaga, T., Wang, J., Kogure, A., Uehori, J., Arase, N., Shiratori, I., Tanaka, S., Kawaguchi, Y., Spear, P. G., Lanier, L. L., Arase, H., PILRalpha is a herpes simplex virus-1 entry coreceptor that associates with glycoprotein B. *Cell* 2008, 132, (6), 935-44.

[63] Wang, J., Fan, Q., Satoh, T., Arii, J., Lanier, L. L., Spear, P. G., Kawaguchi, Y., Arase, H., Binding of herpes simplex virus glycoprotein B (gB) to paired immunoglobulin-like type 2 receptor alpha depends on specific sialylated O-linked glycans on gB. *J Virol* 2009, 83, (24), 13042-5.

[64] Arii, J., Goto, H., Suenaga, T., Oyama, M., Kozuka-Hata, H., Imai, T., Minowa, A., Akashi, H., Arase, H., Kawaoka, Y., Kawaguchi, Y., Non-muscle myosin IIA is a functional entry receptor for herpes simplex virus-1. *Nature* 2010, 467, (7317), 859-62.

[65] Suenaga, T., Satoh, T., Somboonthum, P., Kawaguchi, Y., Mori, Y., Arase, H., Myelin-associated glycoprotein mediates membrane fusion and entry of neurotropic herpesviruses. *Proc Natl Acad Sci USA* 2010, 107, (2), 866-71.

[66] Bender, F. C., Samanta, M., Heldwein, E. E., de Leon, M. P., Bilman, E., Lou, H., Whitbeck, J. C., Eisenberg, R. J., Cohen, G. H., Antigenic and mutational analyses of herpes simplex virus glycoprotein B reveal four functional regions. *J Virol* 2007, 81, (8), 3827-41.

[67] Cairns, T. M., Fontana, J., Huang, Z. Y., Whitbeck, J. C., Atanasiu, D., Rao, S., Shelly, S. S., Lou, H., Ponce de Leon, M., Steven, A. C., Eisenberg, R. J., Cohen, G. H., Mechanism of neutralization of herpes simplex virus by antibodies directed at the fusion domain of glycoprotein B. *J Virol* 2014, 88, (5), 2677-89.

[68] Krawczyk, A., Krauss, J., Eis-Hubinger, A. M., Daumer, M. P., Schwarzenbacher, R., Dittmer, U., Schneweis, K. E., Jager, D., Roggendorf, M., Arndt, M. A., Impact of valency of a glycoprotein B-specific monoclonal antibody on neutralization of herpes simplex virus. *J Virol* 2011, 85, (4), 1793-803.

[69] Oliver, S. L., Xing, Y., Chen, D. H., Roh, S. H., Pintilie, G. D., Bushnell, D. A., Sommer, M. H., Yang, E., Carfi, A., Chiu, W., Arvin, A. M., A glycoprotein B-neutralizing antibody structure at 2.8 A uncovers a critical domain for herpesvirus fusion initiation. *Nat Commun* 2020, 11, (1), 4141.

[70] Wagner, B., Kropff, B., Kalbacher, H., Britt, W., Sundqvist, V. A., Ostberg, L., Mach, M., A continuous sequence of more than 70 amino acids is essential for antibody binding to the dominant antigenic site of glycoprotein gp58 of human cytomegalovirus. *J Virol* 1992, 66, (9), 5290-7.

[71] Ohlin, M., Sundqvist, V. A., Mach, M., Wahren, B., Borrebaeck, C. A., Fine specificity of the human immune response to the major neutralization epitopes expressed on cytomegalovirus gp58/116 (gB), as determined with human monoclonal antibodies. *J Virol* 1993, 67, (2), 703-10.

[72] Speckner, A., Glykofrydes, D., Ohlin, M., Mach, M., Antigenic domain 1 of human cytomegalovirus glycoprotein B induces a multitude of different antibodies which, when combined, results in incomplete virus neutralization. *J Gen Virol* 1999, 80 (Pt 8), 2183-2191.

[73] Meyer, H., Sundqvist, V. A., Pereira, L., Mach, M., Glycoprotein gp116 of human cytomegalovirus contains epitopes for strain-common and strain-specific antibodies. *J Gen Virol* 1992, 73 (Pt 9), 2375-83.

[74] Ye, X., Su, H., Wrapp, D., Freed, D. C., Li, F., Yuan, Z., Tang, A., Li, L., Ku, Z., Xiong, W., Jaijyan, D., Zhu, H., Wang, D., McLellan, J. S., Zhang, N., Fu, T. M., An, Z., Recognition of a highly conserved glycoprotein B epitope by a bivalent antibody neutralizing HCMV at a post-attachment step. *PLoS Pathog* 2020, 16, (8), e1008736.

[75] Ohlin, M., A new look at a poorly immunogenic neutralization epitope on cytomegalovirus glycoprotein B. Is there cause for antigen redesign? *Mol Immunol* 2014, 60, (2), 95-102.

[76] Potzsch, S., Spindler, N., Wiegers, A. K., Fisch, T., Rucker, P., Sticht, H., Grieb, N., Baroti, T., Weisel, F., Stamminger, T., Martin-Parras, L., Mach, M., Winkler, T. H., B cell repertoire analysis identifies new antigenic domains on glycoprotein B of human cytomegalovirus which are target of neutralizing antibodies. *PLoS Pathog* 2011, 7, (8), e1002172.

[77] Spindler, N., Rucker, P., Potzsch, S., Diestel, U., Sticht, H., Martin-Parras, L., Winkler, T. H., Mach, M., Characterization of a discontinuous neutralizing epitope on glycoprotein B of human cytomegalovirus. *J Virol* 2013, 87, (16), 8927-39.

[78] Wiegers, A. K., Sticht, H., Winkler, T. H., Britt, W. J., Mach, M., Identification of a neutralizing epitope within antigenic domain 5 of glycoprotein B of human cytomegalovirus. *J Virol* 2015, 89, (1), 361-72.

[79] Chandramouli, S., Ciferri, C., Nikitin, P. A., Calo, S., Gerrein, R., Balabanis, K., Monroe, J., Hebner, C., Lilja, A. E., Settembre, E. C., Carfi, A., Structure of HCMV glycoprotein B in the postfusion conformation bound to a neutralizing human antibody. *Nat Commun* 2015, 6, 8176.

[80] Liu, Y., Heim, K. P., Che, Y., Chi, X., Qiu, X., Han, S., Dormitzer, P. R., Yang, X., Prefusion structure of human cytomegalovirus glycoprotein B and structural basis for membrane fusion. *Sci Adv* 2021, 7, (10).

[81] Chesnokova, L. S., Hutt-Fletcher, L. M., Fusion of Epstein-Barr virus with epithelial cells can be triggered by alphavbeta5 in addition to alphavbeta6 and alphavbeta8, and integrin binding triggers a conformational change in glycoproteins gHgL. *J Virol* 2011, 85, (24), 13214-23.

[82] Hong, J., Wei, D., Zhong, L., Wu, Q., Chen, K., Zhang, W., Yang, Y., Chen, J., Xia, N., Zhang, X., Chen, Y., Glycoprotein B Antibodies Completely Neutralize EBV Infection of B Cells. *Frontiers in Immunology* 2022, 13.

[83] Zhang, X., Hong, J., Zhong, L., Wu, Q., Zhang, S., Zhu, Q., Chen, H., Wei, D., Li, R., Zhang, W., Zhang, X., Wang, G., Zhou, X., Chen, J., Kang, Y., Zha, Z., Duan, X., Huang, Y., Sun, C., Kong, X., Zhou, Y., Chen, Y., Ye, X., Feng, Q., Li, S., Xiang, T., Gao, S., Zeng, M. S., Zheng, Q., Chen, Y., Zeng, Y. X., Xia, N., Xu, M., Protective anti-gB neutralizing antibodies targeting two vulnerable sites for EBV-cell membrane fusion. *Proc Natl Acad Sci USA* 2022, 119, (32), e2202371119.

[84] Vollmer, B., Prazak, V., Vasishtan, D., Jefferys, E. E., Hernandez-Duran, A., Vallbracht, M., Klupp, B. G., Mettenleiter, T. C., Backovic, M., Rey, F. A., Topf, M., Grunewald, K., The prefusion structure of herpes simplex virus glycoprotein B. *Sci Adv* 2020, 6, (39).

[85] Su, H., Ye, X., Freed, D. C., Li, L., Ku, Z., Xiong, W., Gao, P., Liu, X., Montgomery, D., Xu, W., Espeseth, A. S., Wang, D., Ma, N., Fu, T. M., Zhang, N., An, Z., Potent Bispecific Neutralizing Antibody Targeting Glycoprotein B and the gH/gL/pUL128/130/131 Complex of Human Cytomegalovirus. *Antimicrob Agents Chemother* 2021, 65, (3).

[86] Meng, W., Tang, A., Ye, X., Gui, X., Li, L., Fan, X., Schultz, R. D., Freed, D. C., Ha, S., Wang, D., Zhang, N., Fu, T. M., An, Z., Targeting Human-Cytomegalovirus-Infected Cells by Redirecting T Cells Using an Anti-CD3/Anti-Glycoprotein B Bispecific Antibody. *Antimicrob Agents Chemother* 2018, 62, (1).

[87] Brey, C. U., Proff, J., Teufert, N., Salzer, B., Brozy, J., Munz, M., Pendzialek, J., Ensser, A., Holter, W., Lehner, M., A gB/CD3 bispecific BiTE antibody construct for targeting Human Cytomegalovirus-infected cells. *Sci Rep* 2018, 8, (1), 17453.

[88] Atanasiu, D., Saw, W. T., Cairns, T. M., Eisenberg, R. J., Cohen, G. H., Using Split Luciferase Assay and anti-HSV Glycoprotein Monoclonal Antibodies to Predict a Functional Binding Site Between gD and gH/gL. *J Virol* 2021, 95, (8).

[89] Maertens, J., Logan, A. C., Jang, J., Long, G., Tang, J. L., Hwang, W. Y. K., Koh, L. P., Chemaly, R., Gerbitz, A., Winkler, J., Yeh, S. P., Hiemenz, J., Christoph, S., Lee, D. G., Wang, P. N., Holler, E., Mielke, S., Akard, L., Yeo, A., Ramachandra, S., Smith, K., Pertel, P., Segal, F., Phase 2 Study of Anti-Human Cytomegalovirus Monoclonal Antibodies for Prophylaxis in Hematopoietic Cell Transplantation. *Antimicrob Agents Chemother* 2020, 64, (4).

Chapter 5

Recent Advances in Hepatitis Virus Neutralizing Antibody Research

Mengyuan Zhao
and Minghui Yang*
School of Life Science; Advanced Research Institute of Multidisciplinary Science,
Key Laboratory of Molecular Medicine and Biotherapy, Beijing Institute of Technology,
Beijing, People's Republic of China

Abstract

Hepatitis viruses constitute a significant global health threat, resulting in substantial morbidity and mortality on a global scale. The pursuit of effective therapeutic strategies to combat hepatitis virus infections remains a paramount objective within the realm of medical research. Among the promising candidates, neutralizing antibodies (NAbs) have emerged as noteworthy therapeutic agents due to their capacity to impede viral entry and replication. This chapter provides an overview of recent advancements in the investigation of NAbs targeting various hepatitis viruses, encompassing hepatitis A, B, C, D, and E viruses. Our discourse delves into elucidating the mechanisms underlying neutralization, as well as their practical applications in the therapeutic domain. Additionally, we shed light on the challenges inherent in this research area and delineate the prospective trajectories for future exploration.

* Corresponding Author's Email: yangmh17@bit.edu.cn.

In: Neutralizing Antibodies and their Role in Health and Disease
Editors: Chenguang Shen, Yang Yang and Minghui Yang
ISBN: 979-8-89113-541-3

Introduction

Hepatitis Viruses and Their Global Impact

Viral hepatitis continues to pose a formidable challenge to human health, representing a leading global cause of mortality. The bulk of the global burden of viral hepatitis is attributed to five distinct hepatotropic viruses, namely hepatitis A virus (HAV), hepatitis B virus (HBV), hepatitis C viruses (HCV), hepatitis D (delta) virus (HDV), and hepatitis E viruses (HEV). These viruses can induce both acute and chronic infections [1].

Among the etiological factors contributing to acute viral hepatitis, acute HAV infection stands out as a significant driver of disease burden. In numerous economically disadvantaged regions, such as sub-Saharan Africa and select areas in South Asia, the seroprevalence of hepatitis A antibodies (anti-HAV) can surpass 90% among individuals by the age of 10. Conversely, in affluent regions, the prevalence of anti-HAV remains notably low, with less than 50% of individuals exhibiting seropositivity by the age of 30 [2]. HEV represents another significant contributor to acute hepatitis, with an estimated 3.3 million cases of acute hepatitis arising annually. The hyperendemic spread of HEV genotypes 1 and 2 is observed in numerous countries throughout Central, South, and Southeast Asia. Furthermore, these genotypes are also hyperendemic in East and West Africa, as well as in Mexico [3]. In developed nations, sporadic cases of HEV genotypes 3 and 4 are on the rise. HEV-1, -2, -3, and -4 genotypes can result in acute hepatitis with a self-limiting course or even progress to acute liver failure [4].

However, infections involving HBV, HCV, or HDV are prominent causes of chronic hepatitis, liver cirrhosis, and hepatocellular carcinoma (HCC). In 2019, approximately 296 million individuals were living with chronic HBV infection, while chronic HCV infection posed another pressing global health concern, affecting over 58 million people worldwide. The global prevalence of chronic HBV across all age groups stood at 4.1% in 2019. The highest prevalence was recorded in the Western Pacific region at 7.1%, followed by the African region at 6.5%. Conversely, the European region reported the lowest prevalence at 1.1% [5]. HCV is estimated to afflict around 3% of the global population, with significant geographic variability, ranging from approximately 1.5% in the United States to nearly 15% in Egypt and soaring to 50% in specific age cohorts in Egypt [6]. The estimated global pooled prevalence of HDV is 0.80% in the general population and reaches 13.02% among HBsAg-positive carriers [4].

Over the past decade, our comprehension of the epidemiology of viral hepatitis and associated treatment approaches has advanced substantially. Nevertheless, viral hepatitis continues to claim the lives of over 1.4 million individuals annually. Consequently, viral hepatitis has ascended to the forefront of global health priorities, prompting the implementation of a series of comprehensive public health initiatives. The World Health Organization (WHO) has outlined an ambitious global elimination strategy for viral hepatitis, with the goal of eradicating it as a public health threat by 2030 [7].

Significance of NAbs in Viral infections

Antibodies assume a pivotal role within the adaptive immune response and stand as a cornerstone in the arsenal against infectious diseases. Monoclonal antibodies are secreted by specialized immune cells, plasmablasts, and plasma cells, stemming from activated B lymphocytes [8]. A defining attribute of antibodies lies in their neutralizing capacity, a process that manifests in diverse ways contingent on the viral epitope's characteristics, antibody class, and the infected cell's nature [9].

Various definitions of neutralization exist, with two widely acknowledged formulations. One defines it as "the loss of infectivity resulting from the binding of antibody molecule(s) to a virus particle, typically occurring independently of other factors." The inclusion of complement in rare instances aside, neutralization is primarily evaluated in vitro by co-incubating antibodies, virus particles, and target cells, thereby demonstrating diminished infection. The second definition characterizes neutralization as "the reduction in viral infectivity resulting from antibody binding to the surface of viral particles (virions), thereby obstructing a step in the viral replication cycle occurring prior to virally encoded transcription or synthesis." In the case of enveloped viruses, this blockade transpires prior to virus entry into a host cell, whereas for non-enveloped viruses, it may occur post-entry [10]. The binding of antibody to infected cells, as well as to free virus particles, can mediate several antiviral activities (Figure 1).

Neutralization occurs when a fairly large proportion of available sites on the virion are occupied by antibody, which leads to the inhibition of virus attachment to host cells or interference with the entry (fusion) process. Antibody Fc-mediated effector systems can affect antibody activity against free virus particles in several ways. First, the activation of complement by antibodies that are bound to virus particles and the deposition of complement components on the virion surface can enhance neutralization. Second, complement activation can lead directly to virolysis. Third, Fc and complement receptors can bind antibody- and/or complement-coated virions, which leads to phagocytosis followed by inactivation of the virion in an intracellular compartment of the phagocyte [11]. As shown in Figure 1, activities against infected cells can be mediated by both neutralizing and non-neutralizing antibodies. Antibodies facilitate virus clearance and the elimination of virus-infected cells via Fc-mediated effector mechanisms [12]. The inhibition of viral replication inside cells by the binding of antibodies to viral molecules that are expressed at the membrane of the cells, presumably through signalling mechanisms, has also been described. Antibodies can inhibit the release of viruses from infected cells and the cell-cell transmission of viruses [11, 12].

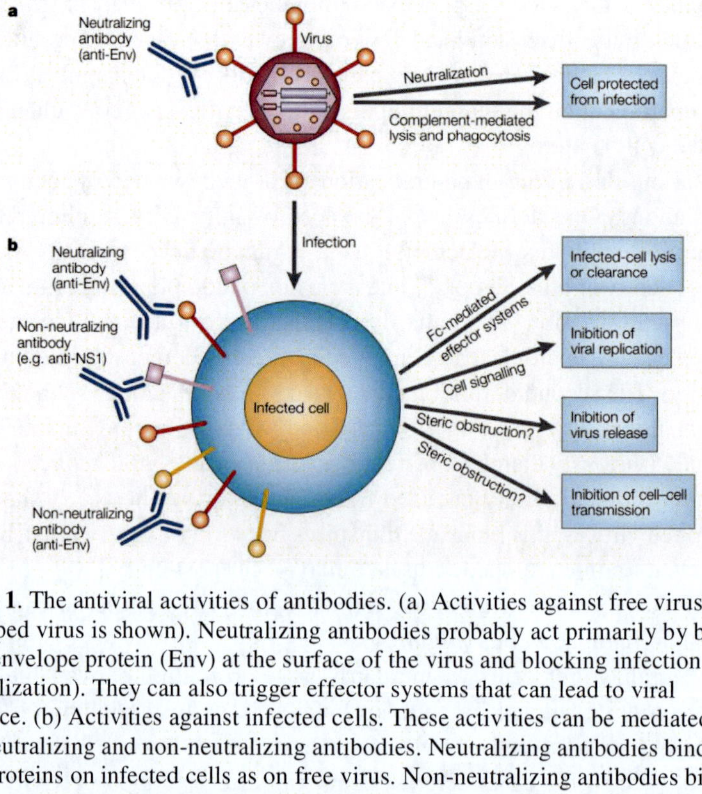

Figure 1. The antiviral activities of antibodies. (a) Activities against free virus (an enveloped virus is shown). Neutralizing antibodies probably act primarily by binding to the envelope protein (Env) at the surface of the virus and blocking infection (neutralization). They can also trigger effector systems that can lead to viral clearance. (b) Activities against infected cells. These activities can be mediated by both neutralizing and non-neutralizing antibodies. Neutralizing antibodies bind to the same proteins on infected cells as on free virus. Non-neutralizing antibodies bind to viral proteins that are expressed on infected cells but not, to a significant degree, on free virus particles. Examples include altered forms of Env protein and certain non-structural (NS) proteins, such as NS1 of dengue virus. Quoted from REF. 11.

NAbs have been demonstrated to impede the viral life cycle at virtually every intracellular stage, ranging from capsid uncoating and endosomal escape to the release of new particles from the infected cell surface [13]. Consequently, NAbs can obstruct infection, eradicate pathogens, and are pivotal in conferring enduring immunity. Capitalizing on these potent antiviral attributes, the transfer of NAbs has emerged as a foundational approach underpinning the utilization of convalescent plasma or plasma-derived immunoglobulins for the prevention and treatment of infectious diseases. Notably, NAbs targeting the capsid proteins of HAV and HEV bestow protective benefits against infection, particularly in the case of HAV, where they can prevent or ameliorate symptoms of acute hepatitis if administered during the initial 2 weeks of the 3- to 4-week incubation phase of infection [14].

Mechanisms of Viral Neutralization

Viral Entry and the Role of NAbs

Viruses, being obligate intracellular pathogens, hinge on their ability to infiltrate host cells, a pivotal phase in their life cycle. Enveloped viruses are encased by a lipid bilayer, while non-enveloped viruses are ensconced within a proteinaceous capsid [15]. Non-enveloped viruses employ various methods, including disrupting the plasma membrane or creating pores, to secure entry. They may also utilize diverse endocytic mechanisms to traverse internal membranes. In contrast, enveloped viruses can either directly fuse with the plasma membrane or navigate the endosomal pathway by traveling in clathrin-coated vesicles, eventually releasing their capsid into the cytosol [16]. Although the strategies employed by non-enveloped and enveloped viruses to traverse membrane barriers differ significantly, both types necessitate specific interactions between host cell molecules or receptors and viral-encoded envelope or capsid proteins [15].

Any antibody displaying sufficient affinity to native structures on virions holds the potential to impede viral entry. A straightforward mechanism of virus neutralization entails obstructing the interaction between virus ligands and cell receptors. Such obstruction can result from antibody binding to the virus ligand or, more commonly, from steric hindrance that interferes with the binding between the virus ligand and the cell receptor [9]. *In vitro*, neutralization mechanisms of enveloped viruses by NAbs encompass

(Figure 2): (a) Preventing the attachment of virions to host cell receptors through disassembly or conformational modification of viral spike proteins. (b) Aggregating virions, hindering their attachment to host cell receptors. (c) Directly impeding the binding of viral spike proteins to host cell receptors through steric interference. (d) Obstructing the fusion of viral and host cell membranes via steric hindrance. (e) Hampering conformational changes in spike proteins necessary for virus entry into host cells. (f) In cases where viruses enter endosomes, impeding entry into the cytoplasm by preventing endosomal cleavage and/or endosomal receptor binding. (g) Blocking viral egress from the cell [10].

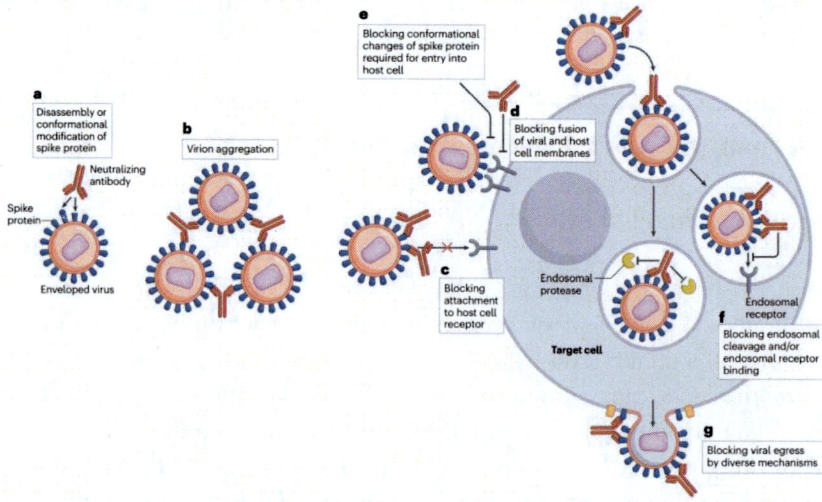

Figure 2. Mechanisms of neutralization of an enveloped virus by neutralizing antibodies *in vitro*. Several mechanisms have been associated with preventing virion attachment to target cell receptors. These include binding to the viral receptor-binding site or in its vicinity and preventing attachment by steric obstruction, disassembling or changing the conformation of viral surface entry proteins, and aggregating virions. NAbs can also interfere with entry post-attachment and have effects post-entry, including in the host cell cytoplasm and during viral egress from host cells. Quoted from REF. 10.

Antibody-Mediated Viral Clearance and Immune Response

A more recently elucidated mechanism of viral inactivation involves antibody-mediated interception of the virus post-entry into the target cell, leading to viral degradation within the cytosol. This process hinges on the recruitment of the intracellular antibody receptor known as TRIM21 [13]. TRIM21 engages with a site located at the interface between the CH2 and CH3 domains within the Fc region of IgG bound to the virus. This interaction culminates in the ubiquitylation of the antibody-bound virus complex, subsequently guiding it to the proteasome for degradation [10]. Notably, this E3 ubiquitin ligase has emerged as a pivotal effector protein, orchestrating intracellular neutralization across multiple viral families. Initially, its role was predominantly associated with non-enveloped viruses. However, recent discoveries regarding TRIM21's involvement in antigen presentation have expanded its significance to encompass enveloped viruses as well [13].

Hepatitis A Virus (HAV)

Epidemiology and Clinical Manifestations

HAV is characterized by a single-stranded, non-enveloped ribonucleic acid (RNA) molecule. It belongs to the *Picornaviridae* family and the *Hepatovirus* genus, primarily transmitted through the fecal-oral route, either via person-to-person contact or the consumption of contaminated food or water sources [17]. Globally, an estimated 1.4 million cases of hepatitis A arise each year, with a relatively low mortality rate of 0.3% [1]. The prevalence of the disease varies significantly across regions and is notably influenced by socioeconomic conditions and access to clean water sources [7]. In regions with inadequate sanitation, the seropositivity for HAV IgG approaches nearly 100% [6].

HAV instigates an acute, self-limiting form of hepatitis that typically resolves spontaneously. The average incubation period spans from 2 to 4 weeks but can extend up to 8 weeks in some cases. Following this incubation period, immune-mediated damage to hepatocytes ensues, leading to nonspecific symptoms such as fever, malaise, fatigue, and loss of appetite. These symptoms are subsequently followed by jaundice, which manifests in approximately 70% of patients [6]. The proportion of asymptomatic infections varies, ranging from 30% in adults to as high as 90% in children under the age of 5. While fulminant hepatic failure is a rare occurrence, it tends to be more prevalent among individuals aged 50 and older, as well as those with preexisting liver conditions. Relapses of acute hepatitis A are observed in 3% to 20% of cases, and in some instances, prolonged or persistent cholestasis may occur post-infection. Importantly, HAV is not associated with chronic infection [1].

NAbs Targeting HAV

The initial evidence of a neutralizing response against HAV came from studies demonstrating the inhibition of focus formation by serum antibodies obtained from both acutely infected humans and nonhuman primates. Notably, the presence of neutralizing antibodies (NAbs) corresponded with a reduction in fecal shedding of HAV in these animals. Further investigations into serum samples from military personnel affected by an HAV outbreak corroborated the existence of a similar neutralizing response to the virus. Through rate zonal centrifugation of serum samples, HAV neutralizing activity was documented in the 7S (IgG) and 19S (IgM) fractions [18]. Moreover, it was observed that the late IgG antibody response exhibited greater efficacy in neutralization compared to the early IgM antibody response [19].

The development of monoclonal antibodies targeting the HAV capsid facilitated the mapping of neutralizing epitopes. In an early study, the RIFA assay and physicochemical methods were employed to partially identify a neutralizing domain within the capsid protein VP1. The use of monoclonal antibodies in cell culture models to select HAV neutralization escape variants expedited the identification of epitopes. These investigations revealed that a predominant conformational (discontinuous) epitope was formed by VP1 and VP3 and was the primary target of NAbs [9]. Another conformational neutralizing epitope was more recently traced to specific amino acid residues within VP2 and VP3, which are targeted by antibodies capable of destabilizing the capsid [20].

HAV Vaccine and Remaining Challenges

Based on well-executed randomized clinical trials involving children in the 1990s, an inactivated HAV vaccine has been licensed and is globally available. Additionally, a live attenuated vaccine is licensed in specific countries, including China, India, Guatemala, the Philippines, and Thailand, with a recommended administration for individuals aged 18 months and older [4].

Comparative large-scale studies from diverse geographic regions evaluating the safety and immunogenicity of both inactivated and live attenuated HAV vaccines are currently lacking. Nevertheless, reports indicate similar safety profiles and efficacy for both types of vaccines. Immunization with a single dose of either the inactivated or live attenuated HAV vaccines results in seroconversion rates exceeding 90% and 94%, respectively [21]. The protective immunity following the initial dose of the inactivated HAV vaccine has been noted to be long-lasting, likely conferring lifelong immunity. Approximately 80% of individuals vaccinated with the live attenuated HAV vaccine still exhibit detectable anti-HAV IgG titers after 15 years. Instances of HAV vaccine immunization failure are exceedingly rare [22].

Given the rising numbers of forcibly displaced individuals in specific regions, endemic HAV infection remains an ongoing but preventable concern necessitating a global response. This response should encompass the provision of public health infrastructure, improved sanitation, and free HAV vaccination programs. Such an approach demands significant collaboration between public health agencies and policymakers alike.

Hepatitis B Virus (HBV)

HBV Infection and Disease Burden

HBV is characterized as an enveloped, partially double-stranded DNA virus, classified within the Orthohepadnavirus genus and further divided into 10 genotypes (A–J). Global estimates provided by the WHO in 2019 disclosed the presence of 296 million HBV carriers, with 1.5 million new infections occurring annually and an annual mortality rate of 820,000 individuals [4]. Chronic HBV infections account for approximately 47% of all deaths related to viral hepatitis, the vast majority of which stem from complications arising from chronic liver disease [7]. Acute hepatitis B manifests between 45 to 180 days following exposure to HBV. The rate of symptomatic infection correlates with age, with less than 10% of children and approximately 50% of adults experiencing symptoms. HBV can persist following acute infection, resulting in chronic hepatitis B infection, a condition inversely associated with age. Fulminant hepatic failure, albeit rare, occurs in up to 1% to 4% of cases, contingent on the patient's clinical background [1].

HBV is highly contagious and spreads through mucous membranes or compromised skin exposed to infected blood or other body fluids such as saliva, semen, and vaginal fluid. Currently, the administration of the hepatitis B vaccine stands as the safest and most effective measure for hepatitis B prevention. Statistical data reveals that 80–95% of the population mounts an immune response following the full course of hepatitis B vaccine inoculation, and its protective efficacy can extend beyond 20 years [23].

NAbs against HBV

Virions and subviral particles prominently exhibit three distinct forms of HBV envelope glycoproteins, collectively known as HBV surface antigen (HBsAg): large HBsAg (L-HBsAg), middle HBsAg (M-HBsAg), and small HBsAg (S-HBsAg). All three forms share a common C-terminal region referred to as the extracellular antigenic loop or major hydrophilic region, which encompasses the immunodominant "a" determinant (amino acids 124-147). This determinant stands as the primary target for antibodies generated in response to both vaccination and HBV infection [24].

Anti-HBs NAbs play a potential role in viral clearance and long-term suppression in individuals who seroconvert to HBV. NAbs elicited by HBV infection typically target the antigenic loop of L-, M-, or S-HBsAg, disrupting attachment to heparan sulfate proteoglycans on hepatocytes. Alternatively, they may target the preS1 domain of L-HBsAg, obstructing binding to the host cellular receptor, the sodium taurocholate cotransporting polypeptide [25]. IgG antibodies directed against the immunodominant "a" determinant of HBsAg, induced through vaccination with recombinant S-HBsAg immunogens, or administered to individuals at risk of exposure via polyclonal Ig infusions, provide protection against HBV infection [26].

Recently, a range of HBV NAbs has been developed and demonstrated efficacy both in vitro and in vivo. These HBV NAbs fall into three major categories: polyclonal antibodies, non-human monoclonal antibodies, and human monoclonal antibodies. Hepatitis B immunoglobulin (HBIG), as a polyclonal antibody, comprises a mixture of antibodies directed against HBsAg. HBIG has been reported to prevent HBV infection, neutralize circulating virions, and induce the lysis of infected cells [27]. However, it is not ideally suited for long-term treatment due to factors such as high cost, limited availability, low specific activity, and the potential risk of infectious agent contamination. These limitations may be overcome through the use of monoclonal NAbs [28].

Monoclonal Antibodies (MAbs) as Therapeutic Agents

Considering the various limitations associated with the clinical use of HBIG, there is potential for the development of HBV-targeting MAbs characterized by high affinity, specificity, and potent neutralizing properties. These MAbs could serve as alternative or complementary products for various applications, including post-exposure prophylaxis for nonimmune individuals, prevention of vertical transmission during childbirth, or the management of HBV recurrence following liver transplantation. In 1984, a murine MAb known as MA18/7 was generated through immunization with purified HBV particles [29]. Additionally, Kucinskaite-Kodze and colleagues generated a panel of murine MAbs designed to target a short linear epitope within the "α" determinant of SHBs. Among these, the HB1 clone exhibited high binding affinity to HBsAg and demonstrated potent HBV-neutralizing capabilities in vitro [30].

However, the therapeutic application of murine MAbs in humans is restricted due to their potential to trigger human anti-mouse antibody (HAMA) responses in patients [31]. With advancements in technology, a new generation of fully human MAbs has been developed, characterized by reduced immunogenicity and improved efficacy, safety, and ease of use. One such example is the human MAb SDZOST577, which targets the "α" determinant of HBsAg and is produced in a hybridoma cell line created by fusing peripheral blood lymphocytes from a healthy adult male vaccinated against hepatitis B with the mouse-human heteromyeloma cell line SPAZ-4. This antibody exhibits high affinity for HBsAg [32]. Furthermore, another fully human MAb, HB-C7A, which also binds to the "α" determinant of HBsAg, has shown significantly greater activity and affinity compared to commercial HBIG [28].

It is worth noting that the administration of a single MAb can exert selective pressure, potentially leading to the emergence of viral escape mutants. Consequently, patients undergoing MAb therapy may develop drug resistance or fail to respond to treatment [33]. To address this concern, a combination of carefully selected MAbs may exert a synergistic effect on neutralization capacity and help prevent the emergence of escape mutants.

Hepatitis C Virus (HCV)

HCV Infection and Chronicity

HCV is a positive-sense single-stranded RNA virus enclosed within an envelope, belonging to the Flaviviridae family. It is currently categorized into 8 genotypes (1–8), with humans serving as the sole natural host for HCV. The incubation period for HCV infection ranges from 14 to 180 days, with only a minority of infected individuals, less than 15%, progressing to acute disease. Among these, approximately 15% experience natural viral clearance, while the rest develop chronic hepatitis C (CHC). CHC is also known to trigger various extrahepatic metabolic and immunologic disorders [1].

Resolution of CHC is associated with the remission of extrahepatic manifestations induced by HCV, and successful HCV clearance may halt the progression of liver disease, potentially even reversing fibrosis and hepatic decompensation [34].

NAbs in HCV Research

The existence of NAbs in the context of HCV infection was first elucidated by Farci and colleagues [35]. The primary targets of NAbs are the HCV envelope glycoproteins (E1 and E2). These glycoproteins are type I transmembrane proteins, highly glycosylated (5-6 and 11 N-glycans, respectively), anchored to the endoplasmic reticulum (ER)-derived membrane via a 30-amino acid transmembrane domain (TMD), and located on the surface of HCV [36].

While both E1 and E2 can serve as NAb targets, the majority of characterized antibodies are directed at E2. Notably, two main immunogenic regions in the E1 protein that induce NAbs have been identified: one located at the N-terminus between amino acids 192–207 and another in the conserved region between amino acids 313–328 near the C-terminus [37]. The human MAb H-111, which targets a linear epitope spanning amino acids 192–202, was isolated from an individual infected with HCV genotype 1b and exhibiting high antibody titers against the E1 glycoprotein [38].

E2 plays an active role in the viral life cycle by facilitating viral entry through interactions with the scavenger receptor-class B type I (SR-BI) and the CD81 receptor [37]. The E2 protein's structure also reveals antigenic regions (AR1-5) and domains (A-E). AR3 holds particular importance in blocking the E2-CD81 interaction [39]. It is a highly conserved region known to induce the generation of broadly neutralizing antibodies capable of inhibiting E2-CD81 binding. This region encompasses the CD81 binding loop and the front layer, earning it the designation of the "neutralizing face" of E2 due to the broadly neutralizing properties of the induced antibodies [40].

Broadly NAbs and Their Potential

The majority of broadly NAbs identified in HCV-infected patients target a conserved antigenic surface referred to as the E2 neutralizing face. This region overlaps with the CD81 receptor binding site and is considered an ideal target for the rational design of an HCV vaccine [40]. The E2 neutralizing face comprises three overlapping neutralizing sites known as antigenic sites AS412, AS434, and AR3 [41].

AS412 represents a conserved region containing two N-glycosylation sites (N417 and N423). Several MAbs directed at AS412 have been extensively characterized, including the mouse MAb AP33 (amino acids 412-423), the human MAb HCV1 (amino acids 412-423), and the mouse MAb24 (amino acids 411-428). Both HCV1 and AP33 MAbs exhibit broad neutralizing capabilities and have demonstrated protection against HCV challenge when passively administered to chimpanzees or mice with a humanized liver, respectively [37].

The MAb 2A5 specifically targets AS434, a conformational epitope situated within the amino acids 434-446 region. This antibody, isolated from a patient with chronic Gt 1b HCV infection, displays neutralization activity against various HCV genotypes and strains in pseudoparticle and cell culture-based HCV systems. Additionally, it has been shown to protect humanized mice from HCV challenges [42].

AR3 (amino acids 523-535) represents another highly conserved region, located within the CD81 binding loop. Due to its pivotal role in the viral entry process through interaction with the CD81 receptor, blocking the E2-CD81 interaction is a central objective of broadly NAbs. Specific MAbs, namely AR3A and AR3B, exhibit the capacity to neutralize pseudotyped HCV particles of genotypes 1a/2a/4/5 in vitro. AR4A, on the other hand, targets the exterior of the CD81-binding site on the E1-E2 complex and can inhibit the entry of cell culture-produced HCV genotypes 1a/1b/2a/3a/4a/5a/6a into host cells in vitro [43].

Some NAbs have been isolated from individuals who spontaneously cleared the infection, as well as from chronic carriers, and have demonstrated broad neutralizing activity. These antibodies offer protection against challenges with both homologous and heterologous HCV strains, and in some cases, they have completely prevented infection [44]. The limitations observed with viral-vectored T-cell vaccines in protecting against progression to chronic hepatitis C suggest that NAbs targeting HCV envelope glycoproteins may play a crucial role in the success of an HCV vaccine. Future hepatitis C vaccine candidates should be designed to elicit a combination of broad humoral and cellular immune responses.

Hepatitis D Virus (HDV)

HDV and Its Unique Characteristics

Hepatitis D infection is caused by HDV, a single-stranded, enveloped RNA molecule. HDV relies on HBsAg for entry into hepatocytes, where it establishes HDV replication. Notably, HDV is the smallest virus known to infect humans and is often classified as a subvirus because its lifecycle is entirely dependent on HBV [45]. Transmission occurs through similar routes as HBV, either concurrently with HBV infection (coinfection) or in individuals with chronic HBV infections (superinfection). Current treatment strategies for HDV primarily focus on prevention and the management of HBV, given that HDV's lifecycle is entirely reliant on HBV. Specific therapies targeting HDV are currently being investigated [6].

NAbs against HDV

In most viral infections, both B- and T-cell immune responses play specific roles in antiviral defense. A successful immune response typically results in either viral elimination or long-term control at low levels. However, for HDV infection, the roles of specific B- and T-cells in either causing liver damage (immunopathogenesis) or eliminating HDV remain unclear. During acute HDV infection, antibodies recognizing both HDV proteins are detected at low titers, which increase significantly during chronic infection [46]. Similar to the immune response to the HBV core antigen, HDV antibodies may not possess the ability to modulate the course of infection and may lack neutralizing activity [47].

Therapeutic Implications and Future Prospects

A recent meta-analysis estimated that approximately 4.5% of individuals positive for HBsAg are coinfected with HDV, translating to approximately 12 million HDV infections globally [48].

Currently, the only available treatment for HDV is interferon, which can affect HDV either through direct inhibition or by targeting HBV. However, numerous trials have demonstrated exceptionally high rates of HDV relapse following interferon therapy [6]. This underscores the urgent need for more effective therapies against HDV. Ongoing research is exploring directed treatments against HDV, including inhibitors of cell entry, prenylation inhibitors, and subviral particle release inhibitors [49].

Hepatitis E Virus (HEV)

HEV Infection and Global Distribution

Hepatitis E infection is caused by the HEV, which is a single-stranded, quasi-enveloped RNA molecule belonging to the Hepeviridae family. There are 8 known genotypes of HEV [6]. HEV genotypes 1 and 2 are responsible for large outbreaks in regions with inadequate sanitation, primarily found in developing countries. These outbreaks are often linked to the consumption of drinking water contaminated with feces. Collectively, HEV genotypes 1 and 2 account for approximately 20.1 million HEV infections, resulting in 3.4 million symptomatic cases, 70,000 deaths, and 3,000 stillbirths each year [7]. Besides infecting humans, HEV genotypes 3 and 4 can also infect various animal species, including swine, deer, and rabbits. These genotypes are more commonly reported in developed countries such as Europe, North America, Australia, and Japan [50]. Transmission of HEV genotypes 3 and 4 is believed to occur through the consumption of undercooked meat, primarily pork [6]. HEV typically causes acute, self-limiting hepatitis, which can be particularly severe in pregnant women. However, cases of chronic hepatitis E have been reported in immunocompromised individuals [1].

NAbs Targeting HEV

The HEV genome is composed of positive-stranded RNA, featuring a short 5' noncoding region and three open reading frames (ORFs) encoding nonstructural proteins (ORF1), capsid proteins (ORF2), and a phosphoprotein (ORF3). The HEV capsid consists of three major domains: S, P1, and P2. Among these, the outermost P2 domain, also known as the E2s domain, appears to be the core antigenic region of the capsid protein, containing crucial neutralization sites responsible for virus-host interactions and NAb induction [51]. For instance, serum collected from an individual with acute HEV genotype 3 infection exhibited high titers of IgM and IgG antibodies that targeted ORF2 and efficiently neutralized virus infectivity derived from stool samples but not from serum [19].

Vaccine Development and Challenges

The capsid protein encoded by ORF2 is considered an ideal candidate for an HEV vaccine. A fragment of the ORF2 capsid protein spanning amino acids 386–606, designated as p239, serves as the minimal unit required for the self-assembly of virus-like particles (VLPs) and has been employed in a highly effective vaccine against HEV infection [19]. Several VLP-based vaccines containing the P2 (E2s) domains have undergone clinical trials. Another recent HEV vaccine candidate, p179, was developed based on the 439-617 region of ORF2 from a genotype 4 strain expressed in *E. coli*. Among these, HEV 239 has been extensively studied, demonstrating its safety and efficacy [4].

However, circulating HEV particles in the blood are quasi-enveloped, making them resistant to antibody-mediated neutralization [19], This resistance poses a challenge for vaccine candidates, as they may lack the efficacy needed to neutralize quasi-enveloped HEV particles. Encouragingly, ongoing research into the function of pORF3 is shedding light on new possibilities for vaccine design against quasi-enveloped HEV particles [52].

Challenges and Future Directions

Immune Escape and Resistance to NAbs

Immune escape, also known as immune evasion or antigenic escape, occurs when the host immune system fails to respond effectively to an infectious agent [53]. This process is observed during the evolution of the virus and aids the virus in its survival [47]. It can reduce the efficacy of vaccines by allowing the virus to evade the host's immune responses. Immune escape mechanisms specific to hepatitis viruses are described below.

In the case of HAV, the effectiveness of the NAb response in preventing the virus's spread in the liver may be limited because the HAV capsid can be cloaked in host cell membranes. Efficient transmission of infection between humans involves naked HAV particles without an envelope component. This envelope protects the virus from IgM or IgG NAbs that block virus attachment or entry at the cell membrane [54]. Quasi-enveloped HAV can be neutralized by IgG after entry into the cell, possibly in the endosome during particle uncoating. Envelope cloaking appears to be an important mechanism for HAV to evade the IgM response that predominates in the early phase of acute infection [19]. Similarly, HEV particles circulating in the blood are quasi-enveloped and resistant to antibody-mediated neutralization. Recent studies have indicated that HEV may employ a second mechanism to evade antibody-mediated neutralization, involving the production of ORF2 capsid protein variants [55].

In the case of HBV, amino acid polymorphisms in viral variants can lead to evasion of neutralization by anti-HBs antibodies induced by the current HB vaccine [4]. Changes in the amino acid sequence within the "a" determinant of the HBsAg can result from point mutations, deletions, or insertions within the S domain of the S-ORF, potentially affecting the binding of NAbs [56].

HCV has developed multiple strategies to avoid recognition by the host's humoral responses. The envelope glycoproteins of HCV are the primary targets of the host's humoral immune response [36]. Studies have demonstrated that humoral immunity exerts selective pressure on HCV, leading to the continuous generation of variants with E1E2 mutations that are not neutralized by circulating NAbs [57]. HCV has also developed other mechanisms to avoid NAb recognition, such as N-glycosylation of HCV E2, which masks epitopes targeted by these antibodies [58]. Additionally, HCV's ability to disseminate using cell-to-cell transmission is an efficient strategy to avoid extracellular compartments where NAbs circulate [59].

Combination Therapies and Novel Treatment Approaches

Over the past decade, significant advancements have been made in diagnosing and managing viral hepatitis, transforming its treatment landscape.

These advances include the development of Direct-acting antivirals (DAAs) for the treatment of chronic HCV, improvements in HBV vaccination, enhanced immunogenicity of HBV vaccines, and the identification of antiviral therapies with low rates of viral resistance [60]. DAAs, in particular, have revolutionized HCV treatment, offering high effectiveness regardless of genotype and a high barrier to resistance. Combinations of DAAs have achieved high sustained virological response (SVR) rates (>95%) with excellent safety and tolerance, even for patients with advanced liver conditions [61]. New drugs targeting HBV, as well as immunomodulatory therapies and gene silencing technologies, are promising approaches to eradicate HBV without harming infected hepatocytes. However, treatment recommendations for acute hepatitis A and E, which are often self-limiting or asymptomatic, are still lacking, even though vaccines have improved prevention. There is an available vaccine for HEV, and clear indications for HAV vaccination now exist [60]. In the case of HDV, effective therapeutic options are currently lacking, necessitating the development of novel targeted antiviral medications that can target HDV cell entry, replication, viral assembly, and release [62].

Despite these advances, challenges related to screening, diagnosis, referral, and treatment of viral hepatitis persist. Nanoparticles have emerged as drug carriers capable of enhancing drug bioavailability and efficacy through drug encapsulation [63]. Additionally, broad vaccination remains crucial. Effective vaccines need to stimulate both arms of the adaptive immune response by inducing early and sustained expansion of specific CD4+ and CD8+ T cell responses alongside the production of cross-reactive NAbs to protect against various variants and genotypes.

Emerging Technologies and Their Impact on Antibody Research

Antibodies are esteemed for their structural integrity, high target affinity, and diverse specificities, making them the foremost natural biological molecules for a wide array of applications. The development of MAbs using hybridoma cell lines marked a significant milestone. Over thirty therapeutic antibodies have been introduced to the market, predominantly in the fields of oncology, autoimmune disorders, and inflammatory conditions [64].

Initially, antibodies were employed as standalone entities, but researchers soon recognized their potential when incorporated into various nanotechnological applications or engineered to create diverse antibody-based modules with enhanced characteristics [65].

Innovations in antibody engineering have opened avenues for designing biobetter antibodies with improved attributes to maximize their efficacy. These enhancements encompass augmenting effector functions, exploring antibody drug conjugates (ADCs), and targeting multiple disease pathways using multi-specific antibodies [66]. Advances in antibody manufacturing processes, including host cell production and purification, are also progressing. Research into the physical and chemical degradation pathways of antibodies is informing the development of more stable proteins, guided by computational tools. Additionally, improvements in the delivery and pharmacokinetics of antibody-based therapeutics are underway, as researchers pursue optimized formulations through recent innovations in the field [64]. For instance, nanoparticles can be custom-designed to target tumor cells in individual patients using MAbs or antibody fragments tailored to specific epitopes unique to the patient's tumor [65]. This approach facilitates precise drug delivery to tumor cells while sparing healthy tissue and minimizing cytotoxic drug-related side effects.

These emerging technologies hold the potential to bring additional advantages to antibody-based strategies for the prevention and treatment of pneumonia viruses.

Conclusion

Recent years have witnessed substantial progress in the study of NAbs against hepatitis viruses. These antibodies not only show promise as therapeutic agents but also enhance our comprehension of viral pathogenesis. Addressing challenges such as viral escape and resistance and developing effective combination therapies are crucial for further advancements. The integration of novel technologies, particularly in the realm of nanotechnology, augurs a bright future for hepatitis virus NAb research, offering the potential for improved treatment and prevention strategies.

References

[1] Lanini, S., A. Ustianowski, R. Pisapia, A. Zumla, G. Ippolito, Viral Hepatitis: Etiology, Epidemiology, Transmission, Diagnostics, Treatment, and Prevention, *Infect Dis Clin North Am*, 33 (2019) 1045-1062.

[2] Jacobsen, K. H., Globalization and the Changing Epidemiology of Hepatitis A Virus, *Cold Spring Harb Perspect Med*, 8 (2018).

[3] Khuroo, M. S., Discovery of hepatitis E: the epidemic non-A, non-B hepatitis 30 years down the memory lane, *Virus Res*, 161 (2011) 3-14.

[4] Elbahrawy, A., H. Atalla, M. Alboraie, A. Alwassief, A. Madian, M. El Fayoumie, A. A. Tabll, H. H. Aly, *Recent Advances in Protective Vaccines against Hepatitis Viruses: A Narrative Review, Viruses*, 15 (2023).

[5] Global, regional, and national burden of hepatitis B, 1990-2019: a systematic analysis for the Global Burden of Disease Study 2019, *Lancet Gastroenterol Hepatol*, 7 (2022) 796-829.

[6] Odenwald, M. A., S. Paul, Viral hepatitis: Past, present, and future, *World J Gastroenterol*, 28 (2022) 1405-1429.

[7] Dunn, R., A. Wetten, S. McPherson, M. C. Donnelly, Viral hepatitis in 2021: The challenges remaining and how we should tackle them, *World J Gastroenterol*, 28 (2022) 76-95.

[8] Imkeller, K., H. Wardemann, Assessing human B cell repertoire diversity and convergence, *Immunol Rev,* 284 (2018) 51-66.

[9] Borrow, P., Mechanisms of viral clearance and persistence, *J Viral Hepat*, 4 Suppl 2 (1997) 16-24.

[10] Burton, D. R., Antiviral neutralizing antibodies: from *in vitro* to *in vivo* activity, *Nat Rev Immunol*, (2023) 1-15.

[11] Burton, D. R., Antibodies, viruses and vaccines, *Nat Rev Immunol*, 2 (2002) 706-713.

[12] Gruell, H., K. Vanshylla, T. Weber, C. O. Barnes, C. Kreer, F. Klein, Antibody-mediated neutralization of SARS-CoV-2, *Immunity*, 55 (2022) 925-944.

[13] Bottermann, M., S. L. Caddy, Virus neutralisation by intracellular antibodies, Semin *Cell Dev Biol*, 126 (2022) 108-116.

[14] Lemon, S. M., J. J. Ott, P. Van Damme, D. Shouval, Type A viral hepatitis: A summary and update on the molecular virology, epidemiology, pathogenesis and prevention, *J Hepatol*, (2017).

[15] Thorley, J. A., J. A. McKeating, J. Z. Rappoport, Mechanisms of viral entry: sneaking in the front door, *Protoplasma*, 244 (2010) 15-24.

[16] Lakadamyali, M., M. J. Rust, X. Zhuang, Endocytosis of influenza viruses, *Microbes Infect*, 6 (2004) 929-936.

[17] Lanini, S., R. Pisapia, M. R. Capobianchi, G. Ippolito, Global epidemiology of viral hepatitis and national needs for complete control, *Expert Rev Anti Infect Ther*, 16 (2018) 625-639.

[18] Lemon, S. M., L. N. Binn, Serum neutralizing antibody response to hepatitis A virus, *J Infect Dis*, 148 (1983) 1033-1039.

[19] Walker, C. M., Adaptive Immune Responses in Hepatitis A Virus and Hepatitis E Virus Infections, *Cold Spring Harb Perspect Med*, 9 (2019).

[20] Wang, X., L. Zhu, M. Dang, Z. Hu, Q. Gao, S. Yuan, Y. Sun, B. Zhang, J. Ren, A. Kotecha, T. S. Walter, J. Wang, E. E. Fry, D. I. Stuart, Z. Rao, Potent neutralization of hepatitis A virus reveals a receptor mimic mechanism and the receptor recognition site, *Proc Natl Acad Sci USA*, 114 (2017) 770-775.

[21] Rao, S., J. S. Mao, S. Motlekar, Z. Fangcheng, G. Kadhe, A review of immunogenicity and tolerability of live attenuated Hepatitis A vaccine in children, *Hum Vaccin Immunother*, 12 (2016) 3160-3165.

[22] Shah, N., M. Faridi, M. Mitra, A. Bavdekar, A. Karadkhele, G. Puppalwar, R. Jain, Review of long term immunogenicity and tolerability of live hepatitis A vaccine, *Hum Vaccin Immunother*, 16 (2020) 2816-2821.

[23] Yang, G., P. Wan, Y. Zhang, Q. Tan, M. S. Qudus, Z. Yue, W. Luo, W. Zhang, J. Ouyang, Y. Li, J. Wu, *Innate Immunity, Inflammation, and Intervention in HBV Infection, Viruses*, 14 (2022).

[24] Bertoletti, A., C. Ferrari, Adaptive immunity in HBV infection, *J Hepatol*, 64 (2016) S71-s83.

[25] Corti, D., F. Benigni, D. Shouval, Viral envelope-specific antibodies in chronic hepatitis B virus infection, *Curr Opin Virol*, 30 (2018) 48-57.

[26] Hehle, V., M. Beretta, M. Bourgine, M. Ait-Goughoulte, C. Planchais, S. Morisse, B. Vesin, V. Lorin, T. Hieu, A. Stauffer, O. Fiquet, J. D. Dimitrov, M. L. Michel, M. N. Ungeheuer, C. Sureau, S. Pol, J. P. Di Santo, H. Strick-Marchand, N. Pelletier, H. Mouquet, Potent human broadly neutralizing antibodies to hepatitis B virus from natural controllers, *J Exp Med*, 217 (2020).

[27] Gaggar, A., C. Coeshott, D. Apelian, T. Rodell, B. R. Armstrong, G. Shen, G. M. Subramanian, J. G. McHutchison, Safety, tolerability and immunogenicity of GS-4774, a hepatitis B virus-specific therapeutic vaccine, in healthy subjects: a randomized study, *Vaccine*, 32 (2014) 4925-4931.

[28] Hong, B., Y. Wen, T. Ying, Recent Progress on Neutralizing Antibodies against Hepatitis B Virus and its Implications, *Infect Disord Drug Targets*, 19 (2019) 213-223.

[29] Heermann, K. H., U. Goldmann, W. Schwartz, T. Seyffarth, H. Baumgarten, W. H. Gerlich, Large surface proteins of hepatitis B virus containing the pre-s sequence, *J Virol*, 52 (1984) 396-402.

[30] Kucinskaite-Kodze, I., M. Pleckaityte, C. M. Bremer, P. L. Seiz, M. Zilnyte, A. Bulavaite, G. Mickiene, G. Zvirblis, K. Sasnauskas, D. Glebe, A. Zvirbliene, New broadly reactive neutralizing antibodies against hepatitis B virus surface antigen, *Virus Res*, 211 (2016) 209-221.

[31] Kunpeng, Z., W. Yugang, C. Jugao, L. Yan, S. Beifen, M. Yuanfang, The construction and expression of a novel chimeric anti-DR5 antibody, *Hybridoma* (Larchmt), 28 (2009) 101-105.

[32] Witherell, G., XTL-001. *XTL Pharmaceuticals, Current opinion in investigational drugs* (London, England: 2000), 3 (2002) 684-692.

[33] Regales, L., Y. Gong, R. Shen, E. de Stanchina, I. Vivanco, A. Goel, J. A. Koutcher, M. Spassova, O. Ouerfelli, I. K. Mellinghoff, M. F. Zakowski, K. A. Politi, W. Pao, Dual targeting of EGFR can overcome a major drug resistance mutation in mouse models of EGFR mutant lung cancer, *J Clin Invest*, 119 (2009) 3000-3010.

[34] Gentile, I., R. Scotto, C. Coppola, L. Staiano, D. C. Amoruso, T. De Simone, F. Portunato, S. De Pascalis, S. Martini, M. Macera, G. Viceconte, G. Tosone, A. R. Buonomo, G. Borgia, N. Coppola, Treatment with direct-acting antivirals improves the clinical outcome in patients with HCV-related decompensated cirrhosis: results

from an Italian real-life cohort (Liver Network Activity-LINA cohort), *Hepatol Int*, 13 (2019) 66-74.

[35] Farci, P., A. Shimoda, D. Wong, T. Cabezon, D. De Gioannis, A. Strazzera, Y. Shimizu, M. Shapiro, H. J. Alter, R. H. Purcell, Prevention of hepatitis C virus infection in chimpanzees by hyperimmune serum against the hypervariable region 1 of the envelope 2 protein, *Proc Natl Acad Sci USA*, 93 (1996) 15394-15399.

[36] Moradpour, D., F. Penin, Hepatitis C virus proteins: from structure to function, Curr Top Microbiol Immunol, 369 (2013) 113-142.

[37] Gomez-Escobar, E., P. Roingeard, E. Beaumont, *Current Hepatitis C Vaccine Candidates Based on the Induction of Neutralizing Antibodies, Viruses*, 15 (2023).

[38] Keck, Z. Y., V. M. Sung, S. Perkins, J. Rowe, S. Paul, T. J. Liang, M. M. Lai, S. K. Foung, Human monoclonal antibody to hepatitis C virus E1 glycoprotein that blocks virus attachment and viral infectivity, *J Virol*, 78 (2004) 7257-7263.

[39] Merat, S. J., R. Molenkamp, K. Wagner, S. M. Koekkoek, D. van de Berg, E. Yasuda, M. Böhne, Y. B. Claassen, B. P. Grady, M. Prins, A. Q. Bakker, M. D. de Jong, H. Spits, J. Schinkel, T. Beaumont, Hepatitis C virus Broadly Neutralizing Monoclonal Antibodies Isolated 25 Years after Spontaneous Clearance, *PLoS One*, 11 (2016) e0165047.

[40] Tzarum, N., I. A. Wilson, M. Law, The Neutralizing Face of Hepatitis C Virus E2 Envelope Glycoprotein, *Front Immunol*, 9 (2018) 1315.

[41] Chen, F., N. Tzarum, X. Lin, E. Giang, R. Velázquez-Moctezuma, E. H. Augestad, K. Nagy, L. He, M. Hernandez, M. E. Fouch, A. Grinyó, D. Chavez, B. J. Doranz, J. Prentoe, R. L. Stanfield, R. Lanford, J. Bukh, I. A. Wilson, J. Zhu, M. Law, Functional convergence of a germline-encoded neutralizing antibody response in rhesus macaques immunized with HCV envelope glycoproteins, *Immunity*, 54 (2021) 781-796.e784.

[42] Desombere, I., A. A. Mesalam, R. A. Urbanowicz, F. Van Houtte, L. Verhoye, Z. Y. Keck, A. Farhoudi, K. Vercauteren, K. E. Weening, T. F. Baumert, A. H. Patel, S. K. H. Foung, J. Ball, G. Leroux-Roels, P. Meuleman, A novel neutralizing human monoclonal antibody broadly abrogates hepatitis C virus infection *in vitro* and in *vivo*, *Antiviral Res*, 148 (2017) 53-64.

[43] Otsubo, R., T. Yasui, Monoclonal antibody therapeutics for infectious diseases: Beyond normal human immunoglobulin, *Pharmacol Ther*, 240 (2022) 108233.

[44] de Jong, Y. P., M. Dorner, M. C. Mommersteeg, J. W. Xiao, A. B. Balazs, J. B. Robbins, B. Y. Winer, S. Gerges, K. Vega, R. N. Labitt, B. M. Donovan, E. Giang, A. Krishnan, L. Chiriboga, M. R. Charlton, D. R. Burton, D. Baltimore, M. Law, C. M. Rice, A. Ploss, Broadly neutralizing antibodies abrogate established hepatitis C virus infection, *Sci Transl Med*, 6 (2014) 254ra129.

[45] Ferenci, P., T. Reiberger, V. Stadlbauer, H. Zoller, Transplantation of hepatitis D virus patients: Lifelong hepatitis B immunoglobulins?, *Liver Int*, (2022).

[46] Fiedler, M., M. Roggendorf, Immunology of HDV infection, *Curr Top Microbiol Immunol*, 307 (2006) 187-209.

[47] Oberhardt, V., M. Hofmann, R. Thimme, C. Neumann-Haefelin, Adaptive Immune *Responses, Immune Escape and Immune-Mediated Pathogenesis during HDV Infection, Viruses*, 14 (2022).

[48] A. J. Stockdale, B. Kreuels, M. Y. R. Henrion, E. Giorgi, I. Kyomuhangi, C. de Martel, Y. Hutin, A. M. Geretti, The global prevalence of hepatitis D virus infection: Systematic review and meta-analysis, *J Hepatol*, 73 (2020) 523-532.

[49] P. Farci, G. Anna Niro, *Current and Future Management of Chronic Hepatitis D, Gastroenterol Hepatol* (N Y), 14 (2018) 342-351.

[50] Zhang, J., J. W. Shih, N. S. Xia, Long-term efficacy of a hepatitis E vaccine, *N Engl J Med*, 372 (2015) 2265-2266.

[51] Aslan, A. T., H. Y. Balaban, Hepatitis E virus: Epidemiology, diagnosis, clinical manifestations, and treatment, *World J Gastroenterol*, 26 (2020) 5543-5560.

[52] Nan, Y., C. Wu, Q. Zhao, Y. Sun, Y. J. Zhang, E. M. Zhou, Vaccine Development against Zoonotic Hepatitis E Virus: Open Questions and Remaining Challenges, *Front Microbiol*, 9 (2018) 266.

[53] Chakraborty, C., A. R. Sharma, M. Bhattacharya, S. S. Lee, A Detailed Overview of Immune Escape, Antibody Escape, Partial Vaccine Escape of SARS-CoV-2 and Their Emerging Variants With Escape Mutations, *Front Immunol*, 13 (2022) 801522.

[54] Feng, Z., L. Hensley, K. L. McKnight, F. Hu, V. Madden, L. Ping, S. H. Jeong, C. Walker, R. E. Lanford, S. M. Lemon, A pathogenic picornavirus acquires an envelope by hijacking cellular membranes, *Nature*, 496 (2013) 367-371.

[55] Yin, X., D. Ying, S. Lhomme, Z. Tang, C. M. Walker, N. Xia, Z. Zheng, Z. Feng, Origin, antigenicity, and function of a secreted form of ORF2 in hepatitis E virus infection, *Proc Natl Acad Sci USA*, 115 (2018) 4773-4778.

[56] Lazarevic, I., A. Banko, D. Miljanovic, M. Cupic, *Immune-Escape Hepatitis B Virus Mutations Associated with Viral Reactivation upon Immunosuppression, Viruses,* 11 (2019).

[57] von Hahn, T., J. C. Yoon, H. Alter, C. M. Rice, B. Rehermann, P. Balfe, J. A. McKeating, Hepatitis C virus continuously escapes from neutralizing antibody and T-cell responses during chronic infection in vivo, *Gastroenterology*, 132 (2007) 667-678.

[58] Helle, F., A. Goffard, V. Morel, G. Duverlie, J. McKeating, Z. Y. Keck, S. Foung, F. Penin, J. Dubuisson, C. Voisset, The neutralizing activity of anti-hepatitis C virus antibodies is modulated by specific glycans on the E2 envelope protein, *J Virol*, 81 (2007) 8101-8111.

[59] Brimacombe, C. L., J. Grove, L. W. Meredith, K. Hu, A. J. Syder, M. V. Flores, J. M. Timpe, S. E. Krieger, T. F. Baumert, T. L. Tellinghuisen, F. Wong-Staal, P. Balfe, J. A. McKeating, Neutralizing antibody-resistant hepatitis C virus cell-to-cell transmission, *J Virol*, 85 (2011) 596-605.

[60] Almeida, P. H., C. E. L. Matielo, L. A. Curvelo, R. A. Rocco, G. Felga, B. Della Guardia, Y. L. Boteon, Update on the management and treatment of viral hepatitis, *World J Gastroenterol*, 27 (2021) 3249-3261.

[61] Asselah, T., N. Boyer, D. Saadoun, M. Martinot-Peignoux, P. Marcellin, Direct-acting antivirals for the treatment of hepatitis C virus infection: optimizing current IFN-free treatment and future perspectives, *Liver Int*, 36 Suppl 1 (2016) 47-57.

[62] Mentha, N., S. Clément, F. Negro, D. Alfaiate, A review on hepatitis D: From virology to new therapies, *J Adv Res*, 17 (2019) 3-15.

[63] Hughes, G. A., Nanostructure-mediated drug delivery, *Nanomedicine*, 1 (2005) 22-30.

[64] Elgundi, Z., M. Reslan, E. Cruz, V. Sifniotis, V. Kayser, The state-of-play and future of antibody therapeutics, *Adv Drug Deliv Rev*, 122 (2017) 2-19.

[65] Hillman, Y., D. Lustiger, Y. Wine, Antibody-based nanotechnology, *Nanotechnology*, 30 (2019) 282001.

[66] Niwa, R., M. Satoh, The current status and prospects of antibody engineering for therapeutic use: focus on glycoengineering technology, *J Pharm Sci*, 104 (2015) 930-941.

Chapter 6

Research Progress on Neutralizing Antibodies against Orthopoxvirus: Insights for Monkeypox Prevention and Treatment

**Mengjun Li*
and Chenguang Shen†**

BSL-3 Laboratory (Guangdong), Guangdong Provincial Key Laboratory of Tropical Disease Research, School of Public Health, Southern Medical University, Guangzhou, People's Republic of China

Abstract

The re-emergence and spread of monkeypox (Mpox) worldwide poses a severe threat to the health and safety of the global population. This outlines the epidemiological characteristics of monkeypox, the pathological features of monkeypox virus, and the immune response following monkeypox infection, which may help raise awareness of monkeypox virus. In addition, it focuses on summarizing the key proteins of variola virus and the current development of neutralizing antibodies, providing a reference for the subsequent development of specific treatments and vaccines for monkeypox.

Keywords: monkeypox virus, Orthopoxvirus, neutralizing antibodies, prevention, treatment

---

* Corresponding Author's Email: limengjun1625@163.com.
† Corresponding Author's Email: a124965468@smu.edu.cn.

In: Neutralizing Antibodies and their Role in Health and Disease
Editors: Chenguang Shen, Yang Yang and Minghui Yang
ISBN: 979-8-89113-541-3

Introduction

Epidemiology

Monkeypox is a zoonotic disease caused by the monkeypox virus and was initially primarily found in Central and West Africa [1]. Since May 2022, confirmed cases of human monkeypox have been reported in several non-endemic countries including the United Kingdom, Spain, Portugal, and China [2]. According to data from the World Health Organization as of July 4, 2023, monkeypox cases have been detected in 112 countries and regions globally, resulting in over 88,144 infections and nearly 150 deaths [3]. Additionally, over 13% of individuals infected with MPXV are asymptomatic, and the symptoms are often atypical, making it easily misdiagnosed as other diseases such as sexually transmitted infections or COVID-19. This increases the risk of hidden transmission of MPXV [4]. Monkeypox virus can be transmitted through contact with infected skin, body fluids, or respiratory droplets, as well as through the exchange of oral and nasopharyngeal secretions or skin-to-skin inoculation, rapidly replicating at the site of inoculation and spreading to nearby lymph nodes [2]. The recent monkeypox outbreaks have mainly occurred in men who have sex with men (MSM) or bisexual men [3], but it is still unclear whether sexual contact directly contributes to the spread of monkeypox [5]. In previous cases of monkeypox virus infection, symptoms included fever, chills, headache, muscle aches, back pain, and fatigue, progressing to exhaustion. The incubation period is usually 7-14 days but can be as long as 21 days. After the onset of fever, the infected individual develops a rash on the face, which then spreads to other parts of the body, starting in the oral and pharyngeal areas and then becoming generalized [6] (Figure 1). Current reports suggest that the disease manifestations in the current outbreak are different from previous ones, as there is no longer a clear distinction between prodromal symptoms and the appearance of skin lesions, and only about half of the cases describe systemic symptoms. In addition, the progression of skin lesions and desquamation are no longer synchronous [7]. Furthermore, severe disease can still occur in specific populations such as children, pregnant women, and immunocompromised individuals. Therefore, despite most cases in the current outbreak being mild in symptomatology, it still poses a significant threat to global health.

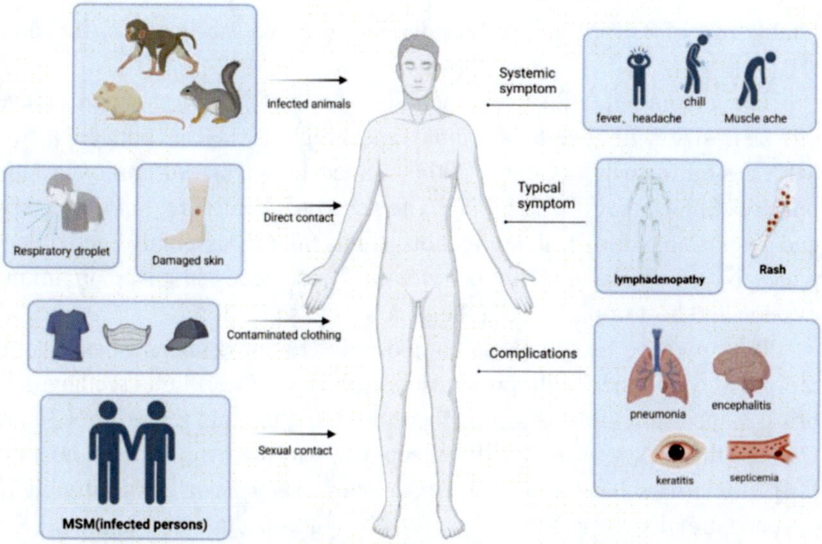

Figure 1. Schematic illustration of the transmission and clinical characteristics of monkeypox. There are many modes of transmission: animals infected with the monkeypox virus (such as squirrels, rodents, and monkeys), direct contact with body fluids or diseased parts of infected animals, scratching or biting by animals, consumption of meat from infected animals, sexual contact (MSM), and contact with contaminated objects, respiratory secretions from those infected individuals, skin lesions, along with their bedding and clothing. The clinical characteristics of monkeypox are depicted on the right side of the figure. Systemic symptoms include fever, headache, chills, muscle aches, and lack of energy—typical symptoms such as lymphadenopathy and rash. Complications of monkeypox include pneumonitis, encephalitis, keratitis, and septicemia. Figure adapted from images created with BioRender.com.

Monkeypox Virus

Monkeypox virus (MPXV) is a member of the Orthopoxvirus genus, including variola, vaccinia, camelpox, and cowpox [8]. MPXV can survive for a long time at 4°C and is resistant to drying. Still, it can be effectively inactivated by organic solvents such as formaldehyde, sodium dodecyl sulfate, methanol, phenol, and chloroform [9]. According to the latest classification by the World Health Organization, MPXV is divided into two lineages: Lineage I (previously known as the "Congo lineage") and Lineage II (previously known as the "West African lineage"). Lineage I is more virulent, with a mortality rate as high as 10.6%, while Lineage II is relatively less virulent, with a case fatality rate of 3.6%. Lineage II is divided into two sub-lineages: IIa and IIb [10, 11].

The genome of MPXV is a double-stranded DNA virus, approximately 197 kb in size, with inverted terminal repeat regions (ITR) at both ends. Some MPXV strains, such as Congo_2003_358, encode over 190 non-overlapping open reading frames (ORFs) [12]. The genome's central region is conserved and responsible for viral replication, transcription, assembly, and release, which is present in all Orthopoxviruses. Most genes involved in immune evasion and host tropism are at the genome ends [12, 13].

The envelope of MPXV is composed of lipoproteins and has a similar morphology to other Orthopoxviruses, typically appearing as rectangular or brick-shaped structures measuring approximately 200 nm × 250 nm × 360 nm. Unlike other DNA viruses, MPXV replicates in the cytoplasm of host cells [14]. Poxviruses have different viral cycles. They enter cells through pH-dependent endocytosis and cell-cell fusion. Intermediate and late viral RNA transcription occurs in the cytoplasm after linear DNA genome replication. They then assemble into non-infectious forms, further processing to generate the first intracellular infectious form of the virus called intracellular mature virus (IMV). Sometimes, virus particles acquire two additional membranes from the trans-Golgi or endosomal membranes, forming intracellular enveloped virus (IEV) or wrapped virus particles. Finally, mature infectious virus particles fuse with the cell membrane and are released as extracellular enveloped virus (EEV) or cell-associated enveloped virus (CEV) [15]. The ability of poxviruses to infect various cells is demonstrated by recruiting numerous proteins. During the replication process, the poxvirus family mainly produces two forms of virus particles: intracellular mature virus (MVs) and extracellular enveloped virus (EVs) [16]. These two forms have different antigens, and the mechanism of poxvirus entry into cells depends on its infectious form. MVs have a single lipoprotein envelope that encloses the virus core and lateral bodies, while EVs have additional membranes and different proteins, which are released through extracellular exocytosis. In addition, MVs are more stable and are believed to mediate transmission between host animals. At the same time, EVs have a fragile outer membrane that allows them to evade host immunity and spread within the host [17-19] (Figure 2). Studies have shown that cowpox virus proteins D8, A27, A34, A26, and H3 are essential in membrane binding and fusion with host cells after virus attachment. Additionally, L1, F9, A28, A27, L5, and H2 are required for virus envelope protein entry into cells [20].

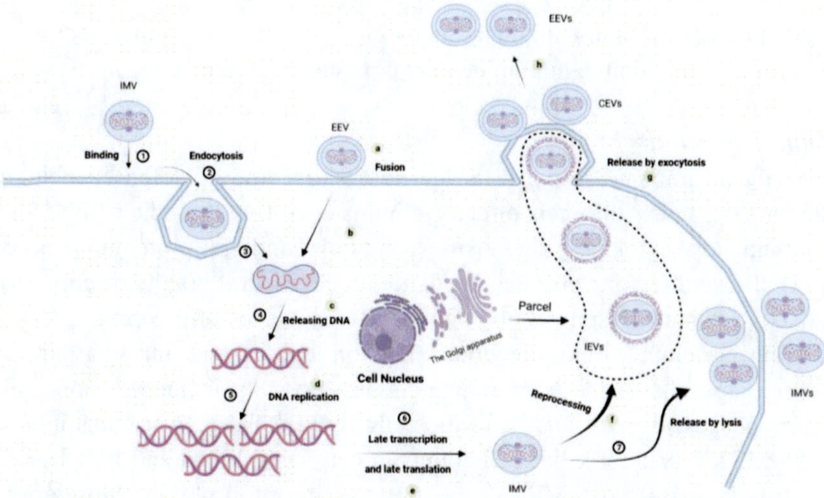

Figure 2. MPXV exhibits typical characteristics of complex orthopoxviruses, with two distinct forms of infection during replication: intracellular mature virion (IMV) and extracellular enveloped virion (EEV). ①-⑦ are the life activities of IMV after entering the host cell. ① IMV binds to the cell surface through movement. ② IMV enters the host cell through endocytosis. ③ After entry, the tegument containing immune modulation proteins disperses. ④ Uncoating occurs, and the core genome is released. ⑤ The released DNA undergoes self-replication. ⑥ Through transcription and translation of late genes, the viral genome is assembled into IMV. ⑦ IMV is released through cell lysis, facilitating the spread between hosts. a-h. are the life activities of EEV after entering the host cell. a. Membrane fusion, EEV enters the host cell through membrane fusion. b-e same as IMV. f. Double membrane wrapping by components from early endosomes or Golgi network forms intracellular enveloped virus particles (IEVs). g. Under the guidance of microtubules, IEVs move towards the cell membrane and attach to the outer layer of the cell membrane, forming cell-associated enveloped virus particles (CEVs). h. CEVs are released from infected cells into the surrounding medium as EEVs, mediating long-distance spread. Figure adapted from images created with BioRender.com.

Immune Response

In research, the interaction between orthopoxviruses and vaccinia virus (VACV) is often used to explain immunity to monkeypox [21]. According to literature reports, non-human primates such as crab-eating macaques and rhesus monkeys have been used to study orthopoxvirus infections, and the pathogenicity of human monkeypox strains from two African lineages has been evaluated in crab-eating macaques. However, the mechanism of systemic or eruptive infection in human monkeypoxes is still unknown [22].

Innate Immunity

The innate immune response is the host's first line of defense, including antiviral proteins that can directly eliminate viruses or induce IFNs, pro-inflammatory cytokines, chemokines, and other antiviral protein expressions [23]. These effector molecules mediate direct antiviral effects or coordinate adaptive immune responses to control different stages of poxvirus infection. During vaccinia virus infection, infection can spread through antigen-presenting cells in the surrounding tissues, possibly including monocytes, macrophages, B cells, and dendritic cells [24]. In rhesus macaques infected with MPXV, natural killer cell counts in peripheral blood and lymph nodes sharply increase. Still, MPXV infection significantly inhibits the migration ability of major subsets of natural killer cells, severely impeding their recruitment to lymph and inflamed tissues [25]. In addition, other innate immune cells, such as macrophages, conventional dendritic cells, plasmacytoid dendritic cells, and innate lymphoid cells, play unknown roles in MPXV-infected patients. Dendritic cells, for example, regulate the function of T cells and influence the growth, differentiation, and function of B cells. During viral infection, DCs are activated by migrating to virus replication and inflammatory sites, such as skin and lungs, to activate immune cells, such as CD8+ T cells, to fight infection and induce immune responses [26].

Adaptive Immunity

The adaptive immune system comprises antigen-specific CD8+ T cells, CD4+ helper T cells, and B cell antibody response, which can provide specificity memory protection against different pathogens [27]. The role of CD4+ T cells in combating viral infections is complex, as they can recruit CD8+ T cells and dendritic cells (DCs), which then activate CD8+ T cells to differentiate into effector and memory T cells, thus promoting B cell-dependent antibody responses [28]. Studies have shown that cytotoxic CD4+ T cells can kill orthopoxvirus-infected cells by inducing perforin in a VACV-infected mouse model, and CD8+ T cells have also been shown to destroy infected monocytes and inhibit viral replication [29, 30]. Furthermore, the quantity of CD4+ T cells is crucial for eliciting protective antibody responses against lethal MPXV infection in vaccinated rhesus monkeys [31]. However, in human studies, there is still no definitive evidence linking CD4+ and CD8+ T cell responses to the severity of MPXV infection [5]. CD8+ T cell responses primarily occur early in infection, while B cells are crucial for antibody production, virus control, and disease prevention later on [32]. VACV-specific B cell responses protect rhesus monkeys from lethal MPXV infection, and VACV vaccines can prevent other poxviruses, including MPXV [33].

Cross-Reactivity and Protective Efficacy of Orthopoxvirus Neutralizing Monoclonal Antibodies Across Species

Mechanism of Neutralizing Antibodies

Neutralizing antibodies (NAbs) can be used for passive immunization and are critical therapeutic agents for rapidly preventing and treating viral infections. Neutralization is the primary mechanism by which antibodies protect against pathogens [34]. Due to their high specificity, good antiviral activity, and low side effects, neutralizing antibodies has become a hot topic in developing antiviral drugs and vaccines.

Neutralizing antibodies, including polyclonal and monoclonal antibodies, protect host cells from pathogen invasion through neutralization or inhibition of the biological effects of the host cells. Polyclonal antibodies, such as convalescent plasma from recovered patients, are mainly used for emergency treatment of viral infections [35]. In contrast, with their high specificity and consistency, monoclonal antibodies have become the preferred tool in many fields.

The mechanism of action of neutralizing antibodies usually involves targeting free viruses and virus-infected cells through a series of mechanisms, including direct blockade of virus entry (neutralization), antibody-mediated effector functions, or indirect blockade of virus entry by crosslinking virus particles to render them inactive (e.g., receptor mimicry). They can also prevent the release of viruses from infected cells or inhibit intercellular spread of the virus (e.g., by avoiding syncytia formation) [36]. The neutralizing mechanisms of the monkeypox virus can be divided into two aspects. On the one hand, for intracellular mature virus (IMV) particles, the current research indicates that the mechanisms of neutralizing antibodies targeting IMV primarily include:

- Blocking virus attachment.
- Preventing IMV penetration into cells.

- Mediating the binding of IMV to cell surface heparan sulfate.

On the other hand, for extracellular enveloped virus (EEV) particles, there is limited research on the neutralizing mechanisms due to the easy destruction of the EEV envelope. It has been reported that inhibition of binding and virus aggregation are among the mechanisms of neutralizing antibodies against EEV [37]. In addition to neutralization, other mechanisms of antibody-mediated protection also contribute to in vivo protection. For enveloped viruses budding from the plasma membrane, antibodies can recruit effector cells or complement, leading to either the killing of infected cells or the lysis of virus particles. Moreover, the same antibodies can inhibit virus assembly, budding, and maturation [34]. Furthermore, non-neutralizing antibodies induced by immunization or infection can protect against viral infection through Fc-mediated effector functions (including antibody-dependent cellular cytotoxicity, opsonization, mast cell activation, and complement activation) [38].

This article focuses on neutralizing antibodies against the monkeypox virus. Previous studies have found that monoclonal antibodies targeting functional proteins of the monkeypox virus can exert potent antiviral effects both in vitro and in vivo. Currently, in mouse infection models, surface proteins A27, L1, H3, D8, A28, A13, and A17 of the monkeypox virus, as well as surface proteins B5 and A33 of the extracellular enveloped virus, have been identified as targets for neutralizing and protective monoclonal antibodies (mAbs) in mice. Additionally, surface protein A10 of the monkeypox virus and surface proteins A56, A34, and A36 of the extracellular enveloped virus may also be potential neutralization targets [39]. Neutralization targets and mechanisms are shown in Table 1. Targeting of MV Particles for Neutralization.

Targeting of MV Particles for Neutralization

The crystal structures of several A27-targeting neutralizing monoclonal antibodies have revealed the structural basis for A27 recognition, which mainly involves the N-terminal region of A27 [40, 41]. It has been found that the binding of A27 and A17 anchors them to the viral membrane, but the specific interaction between them is still largely unclear [42]. Results from Wallengren et al. [43] suggest that the N-terminal domain of A17, displayed on the surface of IMV, serves as an excellent antigenic epitope for neutralizing antibodies. In contrast, the C-terminal domain is located inside the viral membrane. A27, H3, and D8 are glycosaminoglycan (GAG) binding molecules. H3 possesses glycosyltransferase protein folding and binds to UDP-glucose, interacting with cell surface heparan sulfate (HS) during virus entry. It also participates in virus particle morphogenesis and plays a role in infection [44, 45]. Although A27 and H3 bind to heparan sulfate (HS), D8 binds to chondroitin sulfate (CS). The neutralizing monoclonal antibody LA5 against D8 is capable of neutralizing VACV in the presence of complement, indicating that neutralizing antibodies against D8 can block the attachment of the virus to its specific host cells through GAG CS in the presence of complement, thereby exerting neutralization effects [46, 47].

N-myristoylation of L1 is required to form intramolecular disulfide bonds in L1, and neutralizing monoclonal antibodies targeting L1 specifically bind to the native conformation of the intact molecule. If the disulfide bonds of L1 are disrupted, they cannot be recognized by neutralizing antibodies [48, 49]. Ichihashi et al. [50] generated neutralizing antibodies 2D5 and 8C2 against L1, which are capable of inhibiting virus entry and plaque formation. Su et al. [51] found the Fab fragments bound to discontinuous epitopes within L1, composed of two loops linked by a disulfide bond. After cell attachment, L1 mAbs can neutralize VACV, but the neutralization mechanism must be clarified.

A28 and H2 are both components of the entry (or fusion) complex (EFC) of the monkeypox virus, and neutralizing antibodies against the A28 reaction are enhanced explicitly by their association with the H2 protein. The results indicate that the C-terminal region of A28 may contain neutralizing epitopes induced by A28 and H2 immune responses, or proper folding of a conformational epitope is crucial [52].

A13 is one of the few targets that does not participate in binding MV to host cells or entry/fusion, but it plays a critical role in virus particle morphogenesis. Therefore, one possible mechanism by which anti-A13 antibodies neutralize VACV is by generating steric hindrance when they bind to A13 on the surface of virus particles, preventing the attachment and fusion of virus particles with the cell membrane. Another possible mechanism is that anti-A13 antibodies aggregate virus particles by crosslinking A13 on different virus particles [53].

Table 1. List of targeting neutralizing monoclonal antibodies in orthopoxvirus

Activity of netralization	Neutralization Targets	Neutralizing epitope	Neutralization mechanism	References
MV-neutralizing mAbs	L1	disulfide bonds in L1	Preventing viral cell entry and penetration.	[48, 49, 50, 51]
	A27	the N-terminal region of A27	Preventing IMV (Intracellular Mature Virus) penetration into cells.	[40-43]
	A17	the N-terminal region of A17		
	D8	Not available at the moment	In the presence of complement, blocking the attachment of the virus to host cell GAG CS (specifically D8) with specificity.	[46, 47]
	H3	Not available at the moment	Impeding the binding of IMV (Intracellular Mature Virus) to cell surface heparan sulfate.	[44, 45]
	A28	Possibly in the C-terminal region of A28	Obtaining specific enhancement through association with H2 protein.	[52]
	A13	Not available at the moment	Possible generation of spatial hindrance or aggregation of viral particles.	[53]
	A10	Not available at the moment		[39]
EVs-neutralizing mAbs	B5	Not available at the moment	Binding with C1q and C3, resulting in opsonization of viral particles and spatial hindrance to prevent EV (Extracellular Virus) attachment, subsequently leading to CDC (complement-dependent cytotoxicity) upon binding with infected cells.	[56, 57]
	A33	Not available at the moment	Exhibiting protective effects similar to B5 through similar mechanisms.	[65]
	A34	Not available at the moment		[39]
	A36			
	A56			

Targeting of EV Particles for Neutralization

The mechanism of neutralizing antibodies against EV is more complex than against MV, and antibodies targeting EV proteins can prevent viral attacks. Plaque reduction neutralization tests complement fixation inhibition tests, and comet reduction assays neutralize MV and EV [54]. Anti-A33 antibodies induce complement-dependent viral lysis of EV and subsequent release of MV [55]. Neutralizing antibodies against B5 binds to C1q and C3 in a homotypic manner, resulting in the opsonization of viral particles and spatial inhibition of EV attachment to target cells. Simultaneously, binding these antibodies to VACV-infected cells leads to complement-dependent cytotoxicity (CDC), demonstrating adequate protection in both in vitro and in vivo experiments [56, 57]. Two chimpanzee/human monoclonal antibodies with high affinity for B5 and three chimpanzee/human monoclonal antibodies with high affinity for A33 can inhibit comet formation in cowpox virus in vitro, indicating their ability to block virus spread between cells [58-61]. The protective effect of anti-B5 antibodies is not achieved through the traditional direct virus neutralization mechanism because EV is highly tolerant to direct neutralization by anti-B5 antibodies, anti-A33 antibodies, and other EEV targets. However, protective anti-B5 neutralizing antibodies are highly efficient in promoting complement-mediated EEV neutralization, complement-mediated lysis of infected cells, and Fc-dependent protective mechanisms [57, 62-64]. The protective mechanism of A33 antibodies is similar to that of B5 antibodies [65]. Current research suggests that complement enhances the neutralizing effect of monoclonal antibodies and the neutralizing effect of mouse serum immunized with VACV or vaccinated individuals. Still, the role of complement in monkeypox virus (MPXV) activity has yet to be fully elucidated [55, 57, 65].

Cross-Protection by Antibodies and Vaccines

Orthopoxviruses (OPXV), including VARV, VACV, CPXV, MPXV, etc., share more than 90% of their sequence identity between species. All OPXVs encode functionally important homologous proteins involved in entry, gene expression, genome replication, and viral particle assembly. The similarity of structurally expressed proteins among different OPXV explains their immunological cross-reactivity and protective properties [66].

Gilchuk et al. [67] mAbs induced by VACV immunization or MPXV infection targeting any of the six neutralizing determinants (D8, L1, B5 A33, A27, or H3) can inhibit several species of orthopoxviruses. Moreover, the broadest cross-neutralization is primarily mediated by four Abs (LI, D8, B5, H3), and a mixture with different mAb specificities is more effective in achieving neutralization and cross-neutralization. Lei Yang et al. [68] found that antibodies induced by the Vaccinia virus (VACV) Tian Tan strain (VTT) can effectively cross-react with protective antigens of MPXV. In addition, VIG is the only FDA-approved product for treating adverse reactions to VACV vaccination. Due to the common serological cross-reactivity among orthopoxviruses, VIG can react with proteins of other orthopoxviruses, such as MPXV, and has similar therapeutic effects against other poxvirus infections [69, 70].

Based on the initial development against smallpox, the VACV vaccine is now also used to prevent and control monkeypox. Currently, there are three main types of vaccinia virus-based vaccines. The first generation is the live attenuated vaccine, Dryvax, which induces cross-protective immunity against multiple poxviruses. It elicits strong humoral and cellular immune responses and can detect immune responses for several decades after immunization, protecting against the disease for at least 5 years. The second-generation live attenuated vaccine, ACAM2000, is currently approved in the United States for combating monkeypox [71]. ACAM2000 and Dryvax induce specific neutralizing antibodies against VACV regardless of apparent variation in target viral proteins and have been shown to protect against MPXV in animal models [72]. The modified vaccinia virus Ankara Bavarian Nordic (MVA-BN) vaccine is the third generation, highly attenuated virus. Gao et al. [73] MVA can induce specific IgG antibodies against protective antigens of MPXV, neutralize both MVA and current MPXV, and activate cellular immune responses, indicating that the vaccine can effectively cross-react with MPXV.

Conclusion and Outlook

Given the current global epidemic situation of the monkeypox virus and the increasing number of reported cases domestically, it indicates the potential endemic presence of the monkeypox virus in our country. Therefore, comprehensive research on the development, identification, and antiviral mechanisms of monkeypox virus-neutralizing antibodies is of great importance, urgency, and necessity. Referring to the neutralizing targets of orthopoxviruses mentioned above, in our previous studies, our research team immunized mice with a monkeypox-specific protein, A29, which shares homology with A27. Through hybridoma technology, we screened three monoclonal antibodies that recognize different binding epitopes of A29. In both prophylactic and therapeutic protection experiments in animal models, all three antibodies showed efficacy against monkeypox virus infection in mice. Among them, a cocktail of the three antibodies exhibited the best antiviral activity [74]. Considering the current knowledge gap in multifunctional antibodies against orthopoxviruses, developing and identifying highly effective antiviral antibodies against the monkeypox virus have significant scientific research value. Furthermore, current diagnostic techniques for monkeypox are sensitive and relatively complex, with high technical requirements. Therefore, we developed highly sensitive paired antibodies using the "sandwich ELISA" method based on the monoclonal antibodies. We successfully screened paired antibodies with high sensitivity that can detect different poxvirus antigens and specifically detect A29L. Using LIFA technology, we prepared rapid diagnostic kits for both poxviruses and monkeypox-specific antigens [75]. These kits can be used for self-testing at home, as they are easy to operate, safe, require no special equipment, and provide results within 15 minutes, serving as a reference for early diagnosis of monkeypox virus. However, these kits have yet to be applied to clinical specimens for detecting monkeypox infection, and further studies will be carried out to improve their efficacy.

Monkeypox virus has undergone high mutation rates, enabling it to infect new hosts, produce novel virulence factors, evade the human immune system, and spread more rapidly [76]. Currently, no specific therapeutic drugs or vaccines are available for monkeypox, and the neutralizing antibodies discovered so far mainly target the vaccinia virus, with limited research on neutralizing antibodies against monkeypox virus. Moreover, monkeypox virus-specific neutralizing antibodies' epitope recognition and neutralization mechanisms remain unclear and require further investigation.

References

[1] Durski KN, McCollum AM, Nakazawa Y, Petersen BW, Reynolds MG, Briand S, et al. Emergence of Monkeypox — West and Central Africa, 1970–2017. *MMWR*

Morbidity and Mortality Weekly Report: Centers for Disease Control MMWR Office; 2018. p. 306-10.

[2] Kumar N, Acharya A, Gendelman HE, Byrareddy SN. The 2022 outbreak and the pathobiology of the monkeypox virus. *Journal of autoimmunity*. 2022;131:102855.

[3] https://worldhealthorg.shinyapps.io/mpx_global/.

[4] Gispen R, Brand-Saathof B. Three specific antigens produced in vaccinia, variola, and monkeypox infections. *The Journal of infectious diseases*. 1974;129(3):289-95.

[5] Lum FM, Torres-Ruesta A, Tay MZ, Lin RTP, Lye DC, Rénia L, et al. Monkeypox: disease epidemiology, host immunity and clinical interventions. *Nature reviews Immunology*. 2022;22(10):597-613.

[6] Thornhill JP, Barkati S, Walmsley S, Rockstroh J, Antinori A, Harrison LB, et al. Monkeypox Virus Infection in Humans across 16 Countries — April–June 2022. *New England Journal of Medicine*. 2022;387(8):679-91.

[7] Patauner F, Gallo R, Durante-Mangoni E. Monkeypox infection: An update for the practicing physician. *European Journal of Internal Medicine*. 2022;104:1-6.

[8] Xiang Y, White A. Monkeypox virus emerges from the shadow of its more infamous cousin: family biology matters. *Emerging Microbes & Infections*. 2022;11(1):1768-77.

[9] Mukherjee AG, Wanjari UR, Kannampuzha S, Das S, Murali R, Namachivayam A, et al. The pathophysiological and immunological background of the monkeypox virus infection: An update. *J Med Virol*. 2023;95(1):e28206.

[10] Happi C, Adetifa I, Mbala P, Njouom R, Nakoune E, Happi A, et al. Urgent need for a non-discriminatory and non-stigmatizing nomenclature for monkeypox virus. *PLoS biology*. 2022;20(8):e3001769.

[11] Bunge EM, Hoet B, Chen L, Lienert F, Weidenthaler H, Baer LR, et al. The changing epidemiology of human monkeypox-A potential threat? A systematic review. *PLoS neglected tropical diseases*. 2022;16(2):e0010141.

[12] Kugelman JR, Johnston SC, Mulembakani PM, Kisalu N, Lee MS, Koroleva G, et al. Genomic variability of monkeypox virus among humans, Democratic Republic of the Congo. *Emerg Infect Dis*. 2014;20(2):232-9.

[13] Esteban DJ, Hutchinson AP. Genes in the terminal regions of orthopoxvirus genomes experience adaptive molecular evolution. *BMC genomics*. 2011;12:261.

[14] Buller RM, Palumbo GJ. Poxvirus pathogenesis. Microbiological reviews. 1991;55(1):80-122.

[15] Huang Y, Mu L, Wang W. Monkeypox: epidemiology, pathogenesis, treatment and prevention. *Signal Transduction and Targeted Therapy*. 2022;7(1).

[16] Kugelman JR, Johnston SC, Mulembakani PM, Kisalu N, Lee MS, Koroleva G, et al. Genomic Variability of Monkeypox Virus among Humans, Democratic Republic of the Congo. *Emerging Infectious Diseases*. 2014;20(2).

[17] Pickup DJ. Extracellular Virions: The Advance Guard of Poxvirus Infections. *PLoS pathogens*. 2015;11(7):e1004904.

[18] Smith GL, Vanderplasschen A, Law M. The formation and function of extracellular enveloped vaccinia virus. *The Journal of general virology*. 2002;83(Pt 12):2915-31.

[19] Moss B. Poxvirus Cell Entry: How Many Proteins Does it Take? *Viruses*. 2012;4(5):688-707.

[20] Huang Y, Mu L, Wang W. Monkeypox: epidemiology, pathogenesis, treatment and prevention. *Signal Transduct Target Ther*. 2022;7(1):373.

[21] Shafaati M, Zandi M. Human monkeypox (hMPXV) re-emergence: Host immunity status and current vaccines landscape. *J Med Virol*. 2023;95(1):e28251.

[22] Shafaati M, Zandi M. Human monkeypox (hMPXV) re-emergence: Host immunity status and current vaccines landscape. *Journal of Medical Virology*. 2023;95(1).

[23] Gasteiger G, D'Osualdo A, Schubert DA, Weber A, Bruscia EM, Hartl D. Cellular Innate Immunity: An Old Game with New Players. *Journal of innate immunity*. 2017;9(2):111-25.

[24] Stanford MM, McFadden G, Karupiah G, Chaudhri G. Immunopathogenesis of poxvirus infections: forecasting the impending storm. *Immunology and cell biology*. 2007;85(2):93-102.

[25] Song H, Josleyn N, Janosko K, Skinner J, Reeves RK, Cohen M, et al. Monkeypox virus infection of rhesus macaques induces massive expansion of natural killer cells but suppresses natural killer cell functions. *PloS one*. 2013;8(10):e77804.

[26] Lateef Z, Baird MA, Wise LM, Young S, Mercer AA, Fleming SB. The chemokine-binding protein encoded by the poxvirus orf virus inhibits recruitment of dendritic cells to sites of skin inflammation and migration to peripheral lymph nodes. *Cellular Microbiology*. 2010;12(5):665-76.

[27] Medeiros-Silva DC, Dos Santos Moreira-Silva EA, Assis Silva Gomes J, da Fonseca FG, Correa-Oliveira R. CD4 and CD8 T cells participate in the immune memory response against Vaccinia virus after a previous natural infection. *Results in immunology*. 2013;3:104-13.

[28] Sant AJ, McMichael A. Revealing the role of CD4(+) T cells in viral immunity. *The Journal of experimental medicine*. 2012;209(8):1391-5.

[29] Fang M, Siciliano NA, Hersperger AR, Roscoe F, Hu A, Ma X, et al. Perforin-dependent CD4+ T-cell cytotoxicity contributes to control a murine poxvirus infection. *Proceedings of the National Academy of Sciences of the United States of America*. 2012;109(25):9983-8.

[30] Hickman HD, Reynoso GV, Ngudiankama BF, Rubin EJ, Magadán JG, Cush SS, et al. Anatomically restricted synergistic antiviral activities of innate and adaptive immune cells in the skin. *Cell host & microbe*. 2013;13(2):155-68.

[31] Edghill-Smith Y, Golding H, Manischewitz J, King LR, Scott D, Bray M, et al. Smallpox vaccine-induced antibodies are necessary and sufficient for protection against monkeypox virus. *Nature medicine*. 2005;11(7):740-7.

[32] Chaudhri G, Panchanathan V, Bluethmann H, Karupiah G. Obligatory requirement for antibody in recovery from a primary poxvirus infection. *Journal of virology*. 2006;80(13):6339-44.

[33] Jacobs BL, Langland JO, Kibler KV, Denzler KL, White SD, Holechek SA, et al. Vaccinia virus vaccines: past, present and future. *Antiviral research*. 2009;84(1):1-13.

[34] Corti D, Lanzavecchia A. Broadly neutralizing antiviral antibodies. *Annual review of immunology*. 2013;31:705-42.

[35] Shen C, Wang Z, Zhao F, Yang Y, Li J, Yuan J, et al. Treatment of 5 Critically Ill Patients With COVID-19 With Convalescent Plasma. *Jama*. 2020;323(16):1582-9.

[36] Walls AC, Xiong X, Park YJ, Tortorici MA, Snijder J, Quispe J, et al. Unexpected Receptor Functional Mimicry Elucidates Activation of Coronavirus Fusion. *Cell.* 2019;176(5):1026-39.e15.

[37] Law M, Smith GL. Antibody neutralization of the extracellular enveloped form of vaccinia virus. *Virology*. 2001;280(1):132-42.

[38] VanBlargan LA, Goo L, Pierson TC. Deconstructing the Antiviral Neutralizing-Antibody Response: Implications for Vaccine Development and Immunity. *Microbiology and molecular biology reviews: MMBR.* 2016;80(4):989-1010.

[39] Townsend MB, Keckler MS, Patel N, Davies DH, Felgner P, Damon IK, et al. Humoral immunity to smallpox vaccines and monkeypox virus challenge: proteomic assessment and clinical correlations. *Journal of virology*. 2013;87(2):900-11.

[40] Kaever T, Matho MH, Meng X, Crickard L, Schlossman A, Xiang Y, et al. Linear Epitopes in Vaccinia Virus A27 Are Targets of Protective Antibodies Induced by Vaccination against Smallpox. *Journal of virology*. 2016;90(9):4334-45.

[41] Wang D-R, Hsiao J-C, Wong C-H, Li G-C, Lin S-C, Yu SSF, et al. Vaccinia Viral Protein A27 Is Anchored to the Viral Membrane via a Cooperative Interaction with Viral Membrane Protein A17. *Journal of Biological Chemistry*. 2014;289(10):6639-55.

[42] Wang DR, Hsiao JC, Wong CH, Li GC, Lin SC, Yu SS, et al. Vaccinia viral protein A27 is anchored to the viral membrane via a cooperative interaction with viral membrane protein A17. *The Journal of biological chemistry*. 2014;289(10):6639-55.

[43] Wallengren K, Risco C, Krijnse-Locker J, Esteban M, Rodriguez D. The A17L gene product of vaccinia virus is exposed on the surface of IMV. *Virology*. 2001;290(1):143-52.

[44] Davies DH, McCausland MM, Valdez C, Huynh D, Hernandez JE, Mu Y, et al. Vaccinia virus H3L envelope protein is a major target of neutralizing antibodies in humans and elicits protection against lethal challenge in mice. *Journal of virology*. 2005;79(18):11724-33.

[45] Singh K, Gittis AG, Gitti RK, Ostazeski SA, Su HP, Garboczi DN. The Vaccinia Virus H3 Envelope Protein, a Major Target of Neutralizing Antibodies, Exhibits a Glycosyltransferase Fold and Binds UDP-Glucose. *Journal of virology*. 2016;90(10):5020-30.

[46] Matho MH, Maybeno M, Benhnia MR, Becker D, Meng X, Xiang Y, et al. Structural and biochemical characterization of the vaccinia virus envelope protein D8 and its recognition by the antibody LA5. *Journal of virology*. 2012;86(15):8050-8.

[47] Matho MH, Schlossman A, Gilchuk IM, Miller G, Mikulski Z, Hupfer M, et al. Structure-function characterization of three human antibodies targeting the vaccinia virus adhesion molecule D8. *The Journal of biological chemistry*. 2018;293(1):390-401.

[48] Foo CH, Whitbeck JC, Ponce-de-León M, Saw WT, Cohen GH, Eisenberg RJ. The myristate moiety and amino terminus of vaccinia virus l1 constitute a bipartite functional region needed for entry. *Journal of virology*. 2012;86(10):5437-51.

[49] Priyamvada L, Kallemeijn WW, Faronato M, Wilkins K, Goldsmith CS, Cotter CA, et al. Inhibition of vaccinia virus L1 N-myristoylation by the host N-

myristoyltransferase inhibitor IMP-1088 generates non-infectious virions defective in cell entry. *PLoS pathogens*. 2022;18(10):e1010662.
[50] Ichihashi Y, Takahashi T, Oie M. Identification of a vaccinia virus penetration protein. *Virology*. 1994;202(2):834-43.
[51] Su HP, Golden JW, Gittis AG, Hooper JW, Garboczi DN. Structural basis for the binding of the neutralizing antibody, 7D11, to the poxvirus L1 protein. *Virology*. 2007;368(2):331-41.
[52] Shinoda K, Wyatt LS, Moss B. The neutralizing antibody response to the vaccinia virus A28 protein is specifically enhanced by its association with the H2 protein. *Virology*. 2010;405(1):41-9.
[53] Xu C, Meng X, Yan B, Crotty S, Deng J, Xiang Y. An epitope conserved in orthopoxvirus A13 envelope protein is the target of neutralizing and protective antibodies. *Virology*. 2011;418(1):67-73.
[54] Xiao Y, Isaacs SN. Therapeutic Vaccines and Antibodies for Treatment of Orthopoxvirus Infections. *Viruses*. 2010;2(10):2381-403.
[55] Lustig S, Fogg C, Whitbeck JC, Moss B. Synergistic neutralizing activities of antibodies to outer membrane proteins of the two infectious forms of vaccinia virus in the presence of complement. *Virology*. 2004;328(1):30-5.
[56] Benhnia MR, McCausland MM, Laudenslager J, Granger SW, Rickert S, Koriazova L, et al. Heavily isotype-dependent protective activities of human antibodies against vaccinia virus extracellular virion antigen B5. *Journal of virology*. 2009;83(23):12355-67.
[57] Benhnia MR, McCausland MM, Moyron J, Laudenslager J, Granger S, Rickert S, et al. Vaccinia virus extracellular enveloped virion neutralization in vitro and protection in vivo depend on complement. *Journal of virology*. 2009;83(3):1201-15.
[58] McCausland MM, Benhnia MR, Crickard L, Laudenslager J, Granger SW, Tahara T, et al. Combination therapy of vaccinia virus infection with human anti-H3 and anti-B5 monoclonal antibodies in a small animal model. *Antiviral therapy*. 2010;15(4):661-75.
[59] Galmiche MC, Goenaga J, Wittek R, Rindisbacher L. Neutralizing and protective antibodies directed against vaccinia virus envelope antigens. *Virology*. 1999;254(1):71-80.
[60] Chen Z, Earl P, Americo J, Damon I, Smith SK, Zhou YH, et al. Chimpanzee/human mAbs to vaccinia virus B5 protein neutralize vaccinia and smallpox viruses and protect mice against vaccinia virus. *Proceedings of the National Academy of Sciences*. 2006;103(6):1882-7.
[61] Chen Z, Earl P, Americo J, Damon I, Smith SK, Yu F, et al. Characterization of chimpanzee/human monoclonal antibodies to vaccinia virus A33 glycoprotein and its variola virus homolog in vitro and in a vaccinia virus mouse protection model. *Journal of virology*. 2007;81(17):8989-95.
[62] Lustig S, Fogg C, Whitbeck JC, Eisenberg RJ, Cohen GH, Moss B. Combinations of polyclonal or monoclonal antibodies to proteins of the outer membranes of the two infectious forms of vaccinia virus protect mice against a lethal respiratory challenge. *Journal of virology*. 2005;79(21):13454-62.

[63] Vanderplasschen A, Mathew E, Hollinshead M, Sim RB, Smith GL. Extracellular enveloped vaccinia virus is resistant to complement because of incorporation of host complement control proteins into its envelope. *Proceedings of the National Academy of Sciences of the United States of America*. 1998;95(13):7544-9.

[64] Benhnia MR, Maybeno M, Blum D, Aguilar-Sino R, Matho M, Meng X, et al. Unusual features of vaccinia virus extracellular virion form neutralization resistance revealed in human antibody responses to the smallpox vaccine. *Journal of virology*. 2013;87(3):1569-85.

[65] Cohen ME, Xiao Y, Eisenberg RJ, Cohen GH, Isaacs SN. Antibody against extracellular vaccinia virus (EV) protects mice through complement and Fc receptors. *PloS one*. 2011;6(6):e20597.

[66] Moss B. Smallpox vaccines: targets of protective immunity. *Immunological reviews*. 2011;239(1):8-26.

[67] Gilchuk I, Gilchuk P, Sapparapu G, Lampley R, Singh V, Kose N, et al. Cross-Neutralizing and Protective Human Antibody Specificities to Poxvirus Infections. *Cell*. 2016;167(3):684-94.e9.

[68] Yang L, Chen Y, Li S, Zhou Y, Zhang Y, Pei R, et al. Immunization of mice with vaccinia virus Tiantan strain yields antibodies cross-reactive with protective antigens of monkeypox virus. *Virologica Sinica*. 2023;38(1):162-4.

[69] Law M, Pütz MM, Smith GL. An investigation of the therapeutic value of vaccinia-immune IgG in a mouse pneumonia model. *The Journal of general virology*. 2005;86(Pt 4):991-1000.

[70] Lustig S, Maik-Rachline G, Paran N, Melamed S, Israely T, Erez N, et al. Effective post-exposure protection against lethal orthopoxviruses infection by vaccinia immune globulin involves induction of adaptive immune response. *Vaccine*. 2009;27(11):1691-9.

[71] Chakraborty C, Bhattacharya M, Ranjan Sharma A, Dhama K. Monkeypox virus vaccine evolution and global preparedness for vaccination. *International immunopharmacology*. 2022;113(Pt A):109346.

[72] Pugh C, Keasey S, Korman L, Pittman PR, Ulrich RG. Human antibody responses to the polyclonal Dryvax vaccine for smallpox prevention can be distinguished from responses to the monoclonal replacement vaccine ACAM2000. *Clinical and vaccine immunology: CVI*. 2014;21(6):877-85.

[73] Gao F, He C, Liu M, Yuan P, Tian S, Zheng M, et al. Cross-reactive immune responses to monkeypox virus induced by MVA vaccination in mice. *Virology journal*. 2023;20(1):126.

[74] Li M, Ren Z, Wang Y, Jiang Y, Yang M, Li D, et al. Three neutralizing mAbs induced by MPXV A29L protein recognizing different epitopes act synergistically against orthopoxvirus. *Emerging microbes & infections*. 2023;12(2):2223669.

[75] Li M, Wang Y, Li C, Xu R, Chen J, Zhang J, et al. Development of monoclonal antibody-based antigens detection assays for orthopoxvirus and monkeypox virus. *The Journal of infection*. 2022;85(6):702-69.

[76] Reynolds MG, Doty JB, McCollum AM, Olson VA, Nakazawa Y. Monkeypox re-emergence in Africa: a call to expand the concept and practice of One Health. *Expert review of anti-infective therapy*. 2019;17(2):129-39.

Chapter 7

Development of Anti-SARS-CoV-2 Neutralizing Antibodies

Yushan Jiang*
Zihan He
Zhuolin Li
and Chenguang Shen†
BSL-3 Laboratory (Guangdong), Guangdong Provincial Key Laboratory of Tropical Disease Research, School of Public Health, Southern Medical University, Guangzhou, People's Republic of China

Abstract

Variants of severe acute respiratory syndrome coronavirus 2 (SARS-CoV-2) continue to emerge and spread worldwide. Billions of vaccines against SARS-CoV-2 have been administered globally, effectively reducing the morbidity and mortality of coronavirus disease 2019 (COVID-19). The COVID-19 pandemic is wreaking havoc on public health and the global economy. One of the strategies to combat COVID-19 is the development of vaccines with broad-spectrum-neutralizing antibodies for prophylaxis and treatment. Anti-SARS-CoV-2 neutralizing antibodies are important to prevent infections and clear the virus, which is the key to offering long-term immunity. In addition, antiviral antibodies do not always have protective effects. The emergence of SARS-CoV-2 immune escape variants has contributed to the greater importance of vaccine design strategies and antibody-mediated therapies. A few antibodies are currently in preclinical and clinical development,

* Corresponding Author's Email: yushan.y.jiang@gmail.com.
† Corresponding Author's Email: a124965468@smu.edu.cn.

In: Neutralizing Antibodies and their Role in Health and Disease
Editors: Chenguang Shen, Yang Yang and Minghui Yang
ISBN: 979-8-89113-541-3

and a few have been approved for emergency therapy. In this chapter, the current development status of anti-SARS-CoV-2 neutralizing antibodies was reviewed, and the focus was placed on their targets, mechanisms, and taxonomic characteristics. Additionally, severe challenges and possible future directions for neutralizing antibodies were discussed to guide the rational design of next-generation vaccines.

Keywords: SARS-CoV-2, neutralizing antibodies, receptor binding domain, virus mutation, immune evasion

Introduction

The emergence of severe acute respiratory syndrome coronavirus 2 (SARS-CoV-2） disease (COVID-19) has rapidly spread worldwide. As of August 2, 2023, there have been more than 768 million confirmed cases of COVID-19, including more than 6.95 million deaths, reported to WHO [1]. It not only seriously threatens human life and health, but also brings a huge burden to society. The COVID-19 pandemic has been present for over two years [2]. SARS-CoV-2 is an enveloped single-stranded giant RNA virus, which has high nucleotide sequence similarity with Middle East respiratory syndrome coronavirus (MERS-CoV) and severe acute respiratory syndrome coronavirus (SARS-CoV) and belongs to the same group of β-coronaviruses [3]. As it is known, the entry of SARS-CoV-2 into its target cells depends on the binding between the receptor binding domain (RBD) of the viral spike (S) protein and its cellular receptor, angiotensin-converting enzyme 2(ACE2) [4]. Therefore, blocking the binding of S protein to ACE2 is a crucial antiviral intervention.

Neutralizing antibodies are important to fight against viral infections by preventing viruses from entering susceptible cells and blocking the reinfection of newly created offspring. Immediately after the identification of SARS-CoV-2, researchers all over the world embarked on developing neutralizing antibodies against SARS-CoV-2. Antibodies that target the S protein may directly block or effectively interfere with the binding of the virus to the receptor. Thus, most studies have targeted the S protein to find efficient neutralizing antibodies. The Spike (S) protein has two subunits: an N-terminal S1 subunit responsible for receptor binding and a C-terminal S2 subunit responsible for membrane fusion [5]. The S1 protein can be classified into the N-terminal domain (NTD) and the C-terminal receptor binding domain (RBD). RBD is primarily responsible for binding to the receptor [6].

Therefore, targeting the RBD region is the most plausible way to identify potential neutralizing antibodies. Although highly active neutralizing antibodies can also be induced by NTD, the epitopes are typically concentrated in a limited number of similar regions due to the high glycosylation of NTD, resulting in their poor ability to resist many escape mutations of SARS-CoV-2 [7-9]. S2 proteins can also induce neutralizing antibodies and show good broad-spectrum antiviral ability. Nevertheless, the neutralizing activity of these antibodies is generally weak, as the neutralization mechanism of these antibodies does not directly block or interfere with the binding of the virus to the cellular receptors [10, 11]. In contrast, RBD-targeted antibodies with neutralizing activity and broad-spectrum are more suitable for developing antibody candidates against SARS-CoV-2.

This chapter focuses on anti-SARS-CoV-2 neutralizing antibodies. The discovery of neutralizing antibodies, neutralization mechanism and epitope recognition sites of neutralizing antibodies are reviewed in detail. This chapter also proposes current challenges and future directions for neutralizing antibody drug discovery and development. Moreover, recent research on anti-SARS-CoV-2 neutralizing antibodies in recent years is combined to provide an important idea for developing broad-spectrum neutralizing antibodies.

Development and Mechanism of Anti-SARS-CoV-2 Neutralizing Antibodies

Generally speaking, the mechanism of action of most potent neutralizing antibodies involves binding to the RBD, although neutralizing antibodies targeting the NTD domain and the S2 subunit have also been reported [12]. The binding of ACE2 to the RBD of the S protein initiates viral infection [13]. Thus, it is the primary target of neutralizing antibodies. A study of plasma from recovering SARS-CoV-2 patients found that RBD was targeted by 90% of neutralizing antibodies [14]. In the early stage of the COVID-19 pandemic, most studies obtained fully human monoclonal neutralizing antibodies directly from recovered patients or quickly identified candidate antibodies from immunizing animals [15-17]. A study obtained 206 monoclonal antibodies targeting RBD protein and their encoding genes from memory B-cells using recovered patients' peripheral blood mononuclear cells (PBMC) [16] . And was the first to provide a comprehensive overview of antibody responses to SARS-CoV-2, identify highly efficient neutralizing antibodies, and examine their mechanism of action against the virus [16]. Subsequently, Several studies isolated several SARS-CoV-2 RBD antibodies and their sequence features [18-20]. At present, over 5,000 SARS-CoV-2 RBD antibodies have been reported in the world [21, 22]. High-throughput virus neutralization experiments revealed variations in the neutralization activity of RBD antibodies. The bivalent binding of the full-length IgG was found to associate with more RBDs in the "up" conformation than the monovalent binding of Fab, perhaps contributing to the enhanced neutralizing activity of IgG and triggering more shedding of the S1 subunit from the S protein [23]. REGN-COV2 is a cocktail antibody of two recombinant monoclonal neutralizing antibodies: casirivimab (REGN10933) and imdevimab REGN10987) developed by Regeneron Pharmaceuticals [24]. Both antibodies bind the S protein RBD and block its interaction with ACE2 in a simultaneous and non-competitive way. Phase 1-3 trial involving nonhospitalized patients with the original strain of COVID-19 showed reduced viral load, with a greater effect in patients whose immune response had not yet been initiated or who had a high viral load at baseline with good safety [25]. Bamlanivimab (LY-CoV555) is a neutralizing monoclonal antibody (mAb) that binds to the RBD of SARS-CoV-2 S protein and has been shown in Phase II trials to significantly reduce SARS-CoV-2 levels in patients [26]. Etesevimab, or JS016 or LY-CoV016, is a fully human monoclonal neutralizing antibody that binds explicitly to the RBD of SARS-CoV-2 spike protein [27]. Bamlanivimab-etesevimab (LY-CoV016-LY-CoV555) is a cocktail of two antibodies binding to the RBD of the SARS-CoV-2 S-protein, blocking the virus attachment to the human ACE2 receptor, thereby increasing the neutralization rate [28]. Furthermore, various neutralizing antibodies targeting the RBD protein are currently either in clinical trials or in clinical trials worldwide.

The primary mechanism of NTD-targeting neutralizing antibodies may confer protection of conformational changes in S protein and block membrane fusion and viral entry [29]. In addition, 4A8 is the first NTD-targeting neutralizing antibody in the world, with a half-maximal inhibitory concentration (IC50) value of 0.61 μg/mL against the true virus [30]. Other NTD-targeting neutralizing mAbs include COV2-2676, COV2-2489 and DH1050.1 [31, 32]. Of note, the two types of mAbs may be combined to obtain better effectiveness due to the different targets [33]. However, the neutralizing activity of NTD-targeting antibodies is significantly reduced in the face of diverse mutant strains [34].

As the S2 protein of SARS-CoV-2 is crucial for its membrane fusion with cells, it could be targeted by neutralizing antibodies. Nevertheless, the presently S2-targeting antibodies are unsatisfactory and need further investigation [35].

Recognition Sites and Classification Features of Anti-SARS-CoV-2 Neutralizing Antibodies

The SARS-CoV-2 spike protein forms a trimer anchored to the viral membrane, and RBDs exist in two conformational states, described as "up" (open) and "down" (closed) [36]. The ACE2 receptor binding site (RBS) will be exposed only when RBD is in the "up" conformation, which thus mediates the viral invasion of cells. RBS can be effectively recognized by the immune system and induce specific antibodies. RBS occupies a large region of the viral RBD protein, which can be recognized by plenty of antibodies. Additionally, it plays a crucial role in recognizing and binding to the ACE2 receptor. Neutralizing antibodies can approach the viral RBD protein at different angles to target the site or nearby region directly. Owing to the capability of competing with the ACE2 receptor, RBS-targeting antibodies have neutralizing solid activity. Many scholars have proposed that antibodies can be classified according to different recognition epitopes, based on the analysis of antibody structures. The epitope classification of anti-RBD antibodies has been generated by Burton et al., who subdivided RBD-binding antibodies into four classes, i.e., RBS-A, -B, -C, and -D [37]. The non-RBS region of RBD proteins also contains three classes of neutralizing antibody recognition sites, namely S309-, CR3022- and S2H97-site. The recognition sites are distributed on the side of RBD proteins, which results in less competition with the ACE2 receptor [38, 39]. The classification system by Bjorkman et al., divides anti-SARS-CoV-2 RBD antibodies into four epitope classes from classes 1 to 4 [40]. As depicted here, the Class I antibodies described by Barnes et al., as well as the RBS-A and B antibodies of Yuan et al., tend to bind in the area of the peak toward the inner face such as CB6; Class 2 antibodies and RBS-C epitope antibodies like BD-368-2 tend to bind on the outer face of peak area, Class 3 /RBS-D antibodies bind at the lower outer face, also known as the S309 site or the proteoglycan epitope site and typically interact with the glycan attached to residue N343, and Class 4 antibodies such as CR3022 bind on the inner side of the lower part in the area of residues Y369 and S383; Class 5 antibodies represented by S2H97 recognize a new independent epitope and are located "behind" RBD [37]. Recently, Ju et al., isolated 476 S-protein-specific monoclonal antibodies from nine recovered patients infected with the original strain of the SARS-CoV-2 virus. A total of 13 RBD antibodies were able to maintain the ability to neutralize significant mutant strains, like Beta and Delta [41]. However, with the emergence of Omicron mutant strains, seven antibodies remained able to neutralize all mutant strains, suggesting that RBD antibodies could neutralize all mutant strains. In addition, the immunoblot formed by infection with the original SARS-CoV-2 strain could counteract the escape of SARS-CoV-2 mutations. The structural analysis demonstrated that broad-spectrum neutralizing antibodies recognized different epitopes of viruses and could tolerate mutations in their sites of action to a certain extent [42]. The above classification of antibodies based on the different recognition sites of RBD protein is of great significance to understanding antibodies' neutralizing activity and action mechanism.

Challenges of Anti-SARS-CoV-2 Neutralizing Antibodies

SARS-CoV-2 is an RNA virus that undergoes mutations during replication. The S-protein mutation, which first became prevalent and received widespread attention, was D614G. It had no direct contact with RBD-targeting antibodies and no effect on the neutralizing activity of these antibodies. However, SARS-CoV-2 can escape mutations under the selective pressure of antibodies *in vitro* [42]. Zhang et al., elucidated the standard features and characteristics of the "3-53/3-66 public antibodies" of SARS-CoV-2. Furthermore, the authors analyzed the potential for viral mutation escape due to selective pressure from this type of antibodies, suggesting mutations in the K417 site of the SARS-CoV-2 RBD protein could be identified in RBD-targeting antibodies [43]. A study by Cheng et al., investigated the ability of SARS-CoV-2 mutants to escape neutralizing antibodies and their molecular mechanism. It was concluded that SARS-CoV-2 RBD mutations at the K417 site could significantly reduce the neutralizing activity of these antibodies [44, 45]. Nevertheless, Gamma (P. 1) or Beta (B.1.351) strains that carried additional K417 and E484 mutations were capable of significantly escaping from Class 1 and 2 neutralizing antibodies [46]. The emergence of Delta (B.1.617.2) and Kappa (B.1.617.1) strains further increased the ability of viral mutations to escape. L452R mutation led to the partial inactivation of Class 3 neutralizing antibodies [47]. The Lambda mutant (C.37) also escaped Class 3 neutralizing antibodies. It was noteworthy that new mutations like F490S continued to emerge [48]. Most of the mutated strains caused only dispersed or localized epidemics, but the Delta strain triggered a global pandemic because of its high transmission capacity [49, 50]. However, the Omicron variant (B.1.1.529) that suddenly became endemic at the end of 2021 has rapidly replaced the Delta variant as the primary endemic strain worldwide because of its high transmissibility. It was found that the RBD region of the Omicron mutant carries 15 mutation sites capable of significantly escaping the neutralizing effect of antibodies. Among them, K417, E484, G446 and S371 mutation sites mediated the escape of Class 1-4 antibodies, respectively. In particular, mutant strains' first escape of Class 4 antibodies significantly decreased the plasma-neutralizing capacity of CKP survivors and vaccinees [51, 52]. Thus, the emergence of mutation sites in the RBD protein will challenge the development of neutralizing antibodies.

Future Directions for the Development of Anti-SARS-CoV-2 Neutralizing Antibodies

Although the SARS-CoV-2 mutant strain escaped most existing neutralizing antibodies, the neutralizing activity from recovered patients and SARS-CoV-2 vaccines did not wholly disappear. These samples were even able to effectively neutralize the Omicron mutant strain. Suggesting that the original viral infection and vaccines based on original viral sequences could induce a broad spectrum of neutralizing antibodies which can be enriched by the booster immunization of vaccines [53, 54]. STS165, a Class 4 antibody, was isolated from the peripheral blood of a person who recovered from an early epidemic and could neutralize more than 10 variants, including Delta and Omicron [55]. VacW-209, a Class1/4 antibody, was isolated from inactivated vaccine recipients and was also able to efficiently neutralize Omicron and other variants [45, 46]. Moreover, STS165 and VacW-209 could cross-neutralize SARS viruses, demonstrating the broad-spectrum neutralization ability against SARS-CoV-2.

Currently, SARS-CoV-2 continues to mutate. The Omicron mutant variant, which is widely prevalent in the world, has already generated several subclasses, including BA.1, BA.1.1, BA.2, BA.2.12.1, BA.3, BA.4, BA.5, etc. that have substantially escaped from the currently reported antibodies [56, 57]. Conserved epitopes are becoming fewer and fewer with the gradual increase in the number of mutation sites in the RBD region of SARS-CoV-2. Only the recognition region of Class 5 antibodies has not yet undergone the critical escape mutation. This type of antibody can be induced by the natural infection of SARS-CoV-2 and obtained from antigen-immunized mice. This epitope has fewer antibodies in the public domain, such as S2H97, 7D6 and 6D6 [39, 54, 58]. The neutralizing activity of these antibodies is weak, and whether they will escape in the future is unknown. Therefore, developing a new generation of monoclonal broad-spectrum neutralizing antibodies like antibody drug candidates is urgently necessary. According to the action mechanism of RBD-neutralizing antibodies, Class 1 antibodies, which directly block the binding of viruses to the ACE2 receptor, tend to have more robust neutralizing activity. Due to this region's high viral escape frequency, Class 1 antibodies are quickly inactivated by mutations like K417 and ineffective against viral mutations [45, 53, 54]. However, a study by Veesler's group brought hope for developing broad-spectrum neutralizing antibodies with high effectiveness. They isolated S2K146, a monoclonal broad-spectrum neutralizing antibody. S2K146 differs from other published Class 1 antibodies in that it can efficiently neutralize a wide range of SARS-CoV-2 variants and SARS viruses and exhibits ultra-high broad-spectrum properties. Structural analysis revealed the binding of the antibody to viral RBD proteins by mimicking the recognition of the ACE2 receptor [59]. Mutations in the ACE2 region may weaken the binding activity of the virus to the receptor or even lead to the inability to recognize the receptor and make it difficult to survive. Hence, targeting the binding region of the ACE2 receptor may be an ideal target for ultra-broad-spectrum neutralizing antibodies. It is reasonably believed that the discovery of more ultra-broad-spectrum neutralizing antibodies and their structural biology will provide more candidate targets for the future design of neutralizing antibody drugs and broad-spectrum vaccines.

Moreover, exploring better delivery routes and new types of antibodies while actively developing broader-spectrum-neutralizing antibodies will further promote the development and application of SARS-CoV-2. SARS-CoV-2 is transmitted via the respiratory tract, and infection is mainly concentrated in the lungs. Improving the efficiency of antibody delivery to the respiratory tract and lungs is crucial to preventing viral infection, and will help raise antibodies' protective efficiency. It has been demonstrated that SARS-CoV-2 antibodies can be administered by nebulized inhalation and nasal drops in animal models to provide good prevention and treatment of COVID-19 [60, 61]. Regarding the expression form of antibody drugs, traditional antibody drugs are protein-based products with long production cycles and high production costs, which hinder and limit their rapid development and application. Novel mRNA-based antibodies against SARS-CoV-2 are significantly better than traditional protein-based ones in terms of development speed and cost. They can provide longer-lasting protective antibody [62]. Antibody drugs may face the problem of replacement as the current epidemic of SARS-CoV-2 Omicron mutants spreads rapidly and continues to mutate. Besides, mRNA-based antibodies will play a vital role in dealing with the continuous mutation of SARS-CoV-2 by their advantages.

References

[1] WHO. *Coronavirus (COVID-19) Dashboard* [EB/OL] [Available from: Https://covid19.who.int/.

[2] Zhou P, Yang XL, Wang XG, Hu B, Zhang L, Zhang W, et al., A pneumonia outbreak associated with a new coronavirus of probable bat origin (vol 579, pg 270, 2020). *Nature*. 2020;588(7836):E6-E.

[3] Zagaliotis P, Petrou A, Mystridis GA, Geronikaki A, Vizirianakis IS, Walsh TJ. Developing New Treatments for COVID-19 through Dual-Action Antiviral/Anti-Inflammatory Small Molecules and Physiologically Based Pharmacokinetic Modeling. *Int J Mol Sci*. 2022;23(14).

[4] Lu S, Li YG, Ma Q, Nan XF, Zhang ST. A Structure-Based B-cell Epitope Prediction Model Through Combing Local and Global Features. *Frontiers in Immunology*. 2022;13.

[5] Ku ZQ, Xie XP, Davidson E, Ye XH, Su H, Menachery VD, et al., Molecular determinants and mechanism for antibody cocktail preventing SARS-CoV-2 escape (vol 12, 469, 2021). *Nat Commun*. 2021;12(1).

[6] Cusi MG, Di Giacomo AM, Anichini G, Savellini GG, Terrosi C, Gandolfo C, et al., Rational Use of Monoclonal Antibodies as Therapeutic Treatment in an Oncologic Patient with Long COVID. *Viruses-Basel*. 2023;15(3).

[7] Cerutti G, Guo YC, Zhou TQ, Gorman J, Lee M, Rapp M, et al., Potent SARS-CoV-2 neutralizing antibodies directed against spike N-terminal domain target a single supersite. *Cell Host Microbe*. 2021;29(5):819-+.

[8] Graham C, Seow J, Huettner I, Khan H, Kouphou N, Acors S, et al., Neutralization potency of monoclonal antibodies recognizing dominant and subdominant epitopes on SARS-CoV-2 Spike is impacted by the B.1.1.7 variant. *Immunity*. 2021;54(6):1276-+.

[9] McCallum M, De Marco A, Lempp F, Tortorici MA, Pinto D, Walls AC, et al., N-terminal domain antigenic mapping reveals a site of vulnerability for SARS-CoV-2. *Cell*. 2021;184(9):2332-+.

[10] Pinto D, Sauer MM, Czudnochowski N, Low JS, Tortorici MA, Housley MP, et al., Broad betacoronavirus neutralization by a stem helix-specific human antibody. *Science*. 2021;373(6559):1109-15.

[11] Zhou PP, Yuan M, Song G, Beutler N, Shaabani N, Huang DL, et al., A human antibody reveals a conserved site on beta-coronavirus spike proteins and confers protection against SARS-CoV-2 infection. *Sci Transl Med.* 2022;14(637).

[12] Rossotti MA, van Faassen H, Tran AT, Sheff J, Sandhu JK, Duque D, et al., Arsenal of nanobodies shows broad-spectrum neutralization against SARS-CoV-2 variants of concern *in vitro* and *in vivo* in hamster models. *Commun Biol*. 2022;5(1).

[13] Wang XF, Zhang MJ, He N, Wang YC, Yan C, Chen XZ, et al., Potent Neutralizing Antibodies Elicited by RBD-Fc-Based COVID-19 Vaccine Candidate Adjuvanted by the Th2-Skewing iNKT Cell Agonist. *J Med Chem.* 2021;64(15):11554-69.

[14] Piccoli L, Park YJ, Tortorici MA, Czudnochowski N, Walls AC, Beltramello M, et al., Mapping Neutralizing and Immunodominant Sites on the SARS-CoV-2 Spike Receptor-Binding Domain by Structure-Guided High-Resolution Serology. *Cell.* 2020;183(4):1024-+.

[15] Hansen J, Baum A, Pascal KE, Russo V, Giordano S, Wloga E, et al., Studies in humanized mice and convalescent humans yield a SARS-CoV-2 antibody cocktail. *Science*. 2020;369(6506):1010-+.

[16] Ju B, Zhang Q, Ge JW, Wang RK, Sun J, Ge XY, et al., Human neutralizing antibodies elicited by SARS-CoV-2 infection. *Nature.* 2020;584(7819):115-+.

[17] Lv Z, Deng YQ, Ye Q, Cao L, Sun CY, Fan CF, et al., Structural basis for neutralization of SARS-CoV-2 and SARS-CoV by a potent therapeutic antibody. *Science*. 2020;369(6510):1505-+.

[18] Cao YL, Su B, Guo XH, Sun WJ, Deng YQ, Bao LL, et al., Potent Neutralizing Antibodies against SARS-CoV-2 Identified by High-Throughput Single-Cell Sequencing of Convalescent Patients' B Cells. *Cell.* 2020;182(1):73-+.

[19] Robbiani DF, Gaebler C, Muecksch F, Lorenzi JCC, Wang ZJ, Cho A, et al., Convergent antibody responses to SARS-CoV-2 in convalescent individuals. *Nature*. 2020;584(7821):437-+.

[20] Rogers TF, Zhao FZ, Huang DL, Beutler N, Burns A, He WT, et al., Isolation of potent SARS-CoV-2 neutralizing antibodies and protection from disease in a small animal model. *Science.* 2020;369(6506):956-+.

[21] Moriyama S, Anraku Y, Taminishi S, Adachi Y, Kuroda D, Kita S, et al., Structural delineation and computational design of SARS-CoV-2-neutralizing antibodies against Omicron subvariants. *Nat Commun*. 2023;14(1).

[22] Wang YQ, Yuan M, Lv HB, Peng J, Wilson IA, Wu NC. A large-scale systematic survey reveals recurring molecular features of public antibody responses to SARS-CoV-2. *Immunity*. 2022;55(6):1105-+.

[23] Yan RH, Wang RK, Ju B, Yu JF, Zhang YY, Liu N, et al., Structural basis for bivalent binding and inhibition of SARS-CoV-2 infection by human potent neutralizing antibodies. *Cell Res.* 2021;31(5):517-25.

[24] Tada T, Dcosta BM, Samanovic MI, Herati RS, Cornelius A, Zhou H, et al., Convalescent-Phase Sera and Vaccine-Elicited Antibodies Largely Maintain Neutralizing Titer against Global SARS-CoV-2 Variant Spikes. *Mbio*. 2021;12(3).

[25] Liu MT, Gan H, Liang ZM, Liu L, Liu QW, Mai YY, et al., Review of therapeutic mechanisms and applications based on SARS-CoV-2 neutralizing antibodies. *Front Microbiol.* 2023;14.

[26] Shen Q, Li J, Zhang Z, Guo S, Wang QH, An XR, et al., COVID-19: systemic pathology and its implications for therapy. *Int J Biol Sci.* 2022;18(1):386-408.

[27] Ning L, Abagna HB, Jiang QH, Liu SQ, Huang J. Development and application of therapeutic antibodies against COVID-19. *Int J Biol Sci.* 2021;17(6):1486-96.

[28] Kashani NR, Azadbakht J, Ehteram H, Kashani HH, Rajabi-Moghadam H, Ahmad E, et al., Molecular and Clinical Investigation of COVID-19: From Pathogenesis and Immune Responses to Novel Diagnosis and Treatment. *Front Mol Biosci.* 2022;9.

[29] Cao YL, Yisimayi A, Bai YL, Huang WJ, Li XF, Zhang ZY, et al., Humoral immune response to circulating SARS-CoV-2 variants elicited by inactivated and RBD-subunit vaccines. *Cell Res.* 2021;31(7):732-41.

[30] Chi XY, Yan RH, Zhang J, Zhang GY, Zhang YY, Hao M, et al., A neutralizing human antibody binds to the N-terminal domain of the Spike protein of SARS-CoV-2. *Science.* 2020;369(6504):650-+.

[31] Li DP, Edwards RJ, Manne K, Martinez DR, Schäfer A, Alam SM, et al., *In vitro* and *in vivo* functions of SARS-CoV-2 infection-enhancing and neutralizing antibodies. *Cell.* 2021;184(16):4203-+.

[32] Suryadevara N, Shrihari S, Gilchuk P, VanBlargan LA, Binshtein E, Zost SJ, et al., Neutralizing and protective human monoclonal antibodies recognizing the N-terminal domain of the SARS-CoV-2 spike protein. *Cell.* 2021;184(9):2316-+.

[33] Li DP, Sempowski GD, Saunders KO, Acharya P, Haynes BF. SARS-CoV-2 Neutralizing Antibodies for COVID-19 Prevention and Treatment. *Annu Rev Med.* 2022;73:1-16.

[34] Li GY, Qian KW, Zhang SY, Fu WY, Zhao J, Lei CH, et al., Engineered soluble ACE2 receptor: Responding to change with change. *Frontiers in Immunology.* 2023;13.

[35] Yang HT, Rao ZH. Structural biology of SARS-CoV-2 and implications for therapeutic development. *Nat Rev Microbiol.* 2021;19(11):685-700.

[36] Tada M, Aoyama M, Ishii-Watabe A. Characterization of anti-SARS-CoV-2 monoclonal antibodies focusing on antigen binding, neutralization, and FcγR activation via formation of immune complex. *Mabs-Austin.* 2023;15(1).

[37] Strohl WR, Ku ZQ, An ZQ, Carroll SF, Keyt BA, Strohl LM. Passive Immunotherapy Against SARS-CoV-2: From Plasma-Based Therapy to Single Potent Antibodies in the Race to Stay Ahead of the Variants. *Biodrugs.* 2022;36(3):231-323.

[38] Pinto D PY, Beltramello M, Walls AC, Tortorici MA, Bianchi S, Jaconi S, Culap K, Zatta F, De Marco A, Peter A, Guarino B, Spreafico R, Cameroni E, Case JB, Chen RE, Havenar-Daughton C, Snell G, Telenti A, Virgin HW, Lanzavecchia A, Diamond MS, Fink K, Veesler D, Corti D. Cross-neutralization of SARS-CoV-2 by a human monoclonal SARS-CoV antibody. *Nature.* 2020;583(7815):290-5.

[39] Starr TN, Czudnochowski N, Liu ZM, Zatta F, Park YJ, Addetia A, et al., SARS-CoV-2 RBD antibodies that maximize breadth and resistance to escape. *Nature.* 2021;597(7874):97-+.

[40] Barnes CO, Jette CA, Abernathy ME, Dam KMA, Esswein SR, Gristick HB, et al., SARS-CoV-2 neutralizing antibody structures inform therapeutic strategies. *Nature.* 2020;588(7839):682-+.

[41] Ju B, Zhang Q, Wang ZY, Aw ZQ, Chen P, Zhou B, et al., Infection with wild-type SARS-CoV-2 elicits broadly neutralizing and protective antibodies against omicron subvariants. *Nat Immunol.* 2023;24(4):690-+.

[42] Baum A, Fulton BO, Wloga E, Copin R, Pascal KE, Russo V, et al., Antibody cocktail to SARS-CoV-2 spike protein prevents rapid mutational escape seen with individual antibodies. *Science.* 2020;369(6506):1014-+.

[43] Zhang Q, Ju B, Ge JW, Chan JFW, Cheng L, Wang RK, et al., Potent and protective IGHV3-53/3-66 public antibodies and their shared escape mutant on the spike of SARS-CoV-2. *Nat Commun.* 2021;12(1).

[44] Cheng L, Song S, Zhou B, Ge XY, Yu JZ, Zhang MX, et al., Impact of the N501Y substitution of SARS-CoV-2 Spike on neutralizing monoclonal antibodies targeting diverse epitopes. *Virology Journal*. 2021;18(1).

[45] Ju B, Zheng QB, Guo HM, Fan Q, Li TT, Song S, et al., Immune escape by SARS-CoV-2 Omicron variant and structural basis of its effective neutralization by a broad neutralizing human antibody VacW-209. *Cell Res.* 2022;32(5):491-4.

[46] Wang RK, Zhang Q, Ge JW, Ren WL, Zhang R, Lan J, et al., Analysis of SARS-CoV-2 variant mutations reveals neutralization escape mechanisms and the ability to use ACE2 receptors from additional species. *Immunity.* 2021;54(7):1611-+.

[47] Cheng L, Song S, Fan Q, Shen SL, Wang HY, Zhou B, et al., Cross-neutralization of SARS-CoV-2 Kappa and Delta variants by inactivated vaccine-elicited serum and monoclonal antibodies. *Cell Discov*. 2021;7(1).

[48] Guo HM, Fan Q, Song S, Shen SL, Zhou B, Wang HY, et al., Increased resistance of SARS-CoV-2 Lambda variant to antibody neutralization. *J Clin Virol.* 2022;150.

[49] Liu C, Ginn HM, Dejnirattisai W, Supasa P, Wang BB, Tuekprakhon A, et al., Reduced neutralization of SARS-CoV-2 B.1.617 by vaccine and convalescent serum. *Cell*. 2021;184(16):4220-+.

[50] Planas D, Veyer D, Baidaliuk A, Staropoli I, Guivel-Benhassine F, Rajah MM, et al., Reduced sensitivity of SARS-CoV-2 variant Delta to antibody neutralization. *Nature*. 2021;596(7871):276-+.

[51] Cameroni E, Bowen JE, Rosen LE, Saliba C, Zepeda SK, Culap K, et al., Broadly neutralizing antibodies overcome SARS-CoV-2 Omicron antigenic shift. *Nature.* 2022;602(7898):664-+.

[52] Liu LH, Iketani S, Guo YC, Chan JFW, Wang M, Liu LY, et al., Striking antibody evasion manifested by the Omicron variant of SARS-CoV-2. *Nature.* 2022;602(7898):676-+.

[53] Muecksch F, Wang ZJ, Cho A, Gaebler C, Ben Tanfous T, DaSilva J, et al., Increased memory B cell potency and breadth after a SARS-CoV-2 mRNA boost. *Nature*. 2022;607(7917):128-+.

[54] Zhang Z, Ju B, Zhou XR, Cheng L, Wang HY, Liao XJ, et al., The SARS-CoV-2 inactivated vaccine enhances the broad neutralization against variants in individuals recovered from COVID-19 up to one year. *Emerg Microbes Infec.* 2022;11(1): 753-6.

[55] Li YN, Fan Q, Zhou B, Shen YP, Zhang YY, Cheng L, et al., Structural and functional analysis of an inter-Spike bivalent neutralizing antibody against SARS-CoV-2 variants. *Iscience.* 2022;25(6).

[56] Ai JW, Wang X, He XY, Zhao XY, Zhang Y, Jiang YC, et al., Antibody evasion of SARS-CoV-2 Omicron BA.1, BA.1.1, BA.2, and BA.3 sub-lineages. *Cell Host Microbe*. 2022;30(8):1077-+.

[57] Wang Q, Guo YC, Iketani S, Nair MS, Li ZT, Mohri H, et al., Antibody evasion by SARS-CoV-2 Omicron subvariants BA.2.12.1, BA.4 and BA.5. *Nature.* 2022;608(7923):603-+.

[58] Li TT, Xue WH, Zheng QB, Song S, Yang CL, Xiong HL, et al., Cross-neutralizing antibodies bind a SARS-CoV-2 cryptic site and resist circulating variants. *Nat Commun*. 2021;12(1).

[59] Park YJ, De Marco A, Starr TN, Liu ZM, Pinto D, Walls AC, et al., Antibody-mediated broad sarbecovirus neutralization through ACE2 molecular mimicry. *Science.* 2022;375(6579):449-+.

[60] Li C, Zhan WQ, Yang ZL, Tu C, Hu GW, Zhang X, et al., Broad neutralization of SARS-CoV-2 variants by an inhalable bispecific single-domain antibody. *Cell.* 2022;185(8):1389-+.

[61] Lu J, Yin QL, Pei RJ, Zhang Q, Qu YY, Pan YB, et al., Nasal delivery of broadly neutralizing antibodies protects mice from lethal challenge with SARS-CoV-2 delta and omicron variants. *Virol Sin*. 2022;37(2):238-47.

[62] Deng YQ, Zhang NN, Zhang YF, Zhong X, Xu SE, Qiu HY, et al., Lipid nanoparticle-encapsulated mRNA antibody provides long-term protection against SARS-CoV-2 in mice and hamsters. *Cell Res*. 2022;32(4):375-82.

Chapter 8

A Possible Treatment Option for COVID-19: The Inflammatory Factor Antibodies

Jiayang Wang* **and Chenguang Shen†**

BSL-3 Laboratory (Guangdong), Guangdong Provincial Key Laboratory of Tropical Disease Research, School of Public Health, Southern Medical University, Guangzhou, People's Republic of China

Abstract

This chapter discusses the systemic inflammatory pathway in severe COVID-19 patients and explores whether the inflammatory factor antibodies could be a therapeutic option for severe COVID-19 patients. As IL-6 and IFN-γ are the critical factors in systemic inflammatory reactions, the relevant antibodies are potential choices.

Keywords: cytokine storm, COVID-19, inflammatory factor antibodies

Introduction

COVID-19, caused by SARS-CoV-2, has been reported in over 768 million cases and over 6.9 million deaths globally. As the SARS-CoV-2 continually evolves more and more subvariants and the pressure of immune escape grows, the stockpiling of more therapeutic options is one solution to the future. The

---

* Corresponding Author's Email: 742693591@qq.com.
† Corresponding Author's Email: a124965468@smu.edu.cn.

In: Neutralizing Antibodies and their Role in Health and Disease
Editors: Chenguang Shen, Yang Yang and Minghui Yang
ISBN: 979-8-89113-541-3

data from autopsy and clinical indicators shows that the systemic inflammatory reaction is the essential procedure that will cause severe COVID-19, meaning that the patients suffer from respiratory failure, hypoxemia, and even death [1]. One critical cause of severe COVID-19 is a systemic inflammatory reaction, an overactive inflammation sweeps the whole body, causing multiple organ damages. When the immune system fails to clear the virus and becomes dysfunctional, the excess of cytokine becomes harmful to organs, called a cytokine storm.

Thus, the anti-inflammatory treatment plays a vital role in clinical. The inflammatory factor antibodies have great potential to deal with the situation. This chapter will introduce some inflammatory pathways and conclude some antibodies that anti the key inflammatory factors and discuss the possibility of clinical application.

Systemic Inflammatory Reaction in COVID-19

Studies have shown that systemic inflammatory reactions and high mortality are related to cytokine storms. The level of many factors in the blood of severe COVID-19 patients can detected as significantly elevated, such as IL-1, IL-2 IL-6, IL-7, IFN-γ, IFN-γ-induced protein 10(IP10), IFN-1β, TNF-α [2]. Severe COVID-19 patients admitted to the intensive care unit (ICU) can be detected with higher levels of IL-6 and IL-7. IL-10 and IFN-γ [3, 4]. All this evidence suggests severe COVID-19 mortality might be due to cytokine storm.

The concept that overactive inflammation can seriously damage organs and cause rapid clinical deterioration is not a new theory. As severe acute respiratory syndrome (SARS), the first time out broke in Guangdong, China, in 2003. Chinese doctors have already noticed that the pathology of this virus disease was a high-level inflammatory reaction and used glucocorticoids to cure the disease. The cytokine storm caused by immune disorders is called macrophage activation syndrome (MAS) or cytokine release syndrome (CRS).

A study revealed that the reason for cytokine storms is the failure of the immune system to clear the virus. The whole procedure can be divided into two stages. The first stage is a temporary immune-deficient condition, and the following stage is an overactive immune situation, accompanied by severe clinical symptoms [5]. Animal experiments have demonstrated that the secretion of type Ⅰ and Ⅲ IFN besides IFN α and IFN β in the early infectious stages, and secretion of pro-inflammatory cytokines from mononuclear macrophages initiates cytokine storm [6]. In addition, the high reaction of inflammatory responses is caused by IL-6 and TNF-α. Studies have shown that non-survivors of COVID-19 have higher IL-6 levels than survivors, and IL-6 is a risk factor for the prognosis of COVID-19. A cohort study demonstrated that high IL-6 and d-dimer are related to thrombotic conditions and predict the mortality of COVID-19 patients in hospitals [7].

In conjunction with these studies, the etiology of acute respiratory distress syndrome (ARDS) in severe COVID-19 patients can be elucidated. Once the immune system fails to clear the virus, the immune cells secrete pro-inflammatory factors like IL-6 and INF-γ and induce chain reactions to cytokine storm and systemic inflammatory reaction, which results in blood clots, vascular damage, olfactory dysfunction, and gastrointestinal symptoms [8]. These pathological conditions worsen the elderly patients who already have underlying disease and cause high mortality of severe COVID-19.

Anti IL-1 Antibodies

IL-1 is an essential pro-inflammatory cytokine that plays an initial role in the immune response. IL-1 has two forms, IL-1α and IL-1β, in which IL-1β has more systemic effects [9]. IL-1 can be secreted by many immune cells such as macrophages and monocytes. IL-1 can recruit more immune cells and activate the subsequent immune response. Through this mechanism, using an inhibitor of IL-1 could benefit patients with COVID-19, improve the outcome of the disease, and reduce the mortality of those in the ICU.

Canakinumab is a human monoclonal antibody targeting IL-1β. It was approved by the FDA in 2009 for curing cryopyrin-associated periodic syndromes [10]. Canakinumab is now used for rheumatoid arthritis, systemic-onset juvenile idiopathic arthritis, chronic obstructive pulmonary disease, type 1 and 2 diabetes, and ocular disease with the advantage of being good-tolerated in patients [11]. Although canakinumab is not for infectious diseases, there is evidence that canakinumab is beneficial to COVID-19 patients because it inhibits the same IL-1 pathway of auto-inflammatory disease. One study has shown that blocking the IL-1 signal in the early stage of COVID-19 would reduce admission to the ICU [12]. One meta-analysis sorted 6 studies, 1121 adults with COVID-19, which revealed that canakinumab treatment could reduce overall mortality and C reaction protein, suggesting lower inflammatory levels [13]. Meanwhile, canakinumab has a good effect on moderate patients, not only on severe patients. One prospective study collected

33 patients who were diagnosed with moderate COVID-19. The canakinumab treatment group rapidly recovered oxygen levels, decreased the rate of invasive mechanical ventilation, and shortened hospital stays [14]. Those patients who already have a chronic disease like diabetes are mostly regarded as high risk for severe conditions. Canakinumab could have a double beneficial effect on these patients because canakinumab was initially used for diabetes. Patients with type 2 diabetes and obesity were associated with chronic inflammatory conditions, which would worsen COVID-19. A double-blind, placebo-controlled trial study made a comparison of canakinumab and placebo. The results suggested that canakinumab could shorten ICU and ventilation time, and type 2 diabetes patients required fewer antidiabetic drugs. The patients whose BMI was higher than 35 kg/m2 would have more benefits, and the inflammatory markers in blood were lower. However, canakinumab didn't improve survival time or length of hospitalization [15].

Anti IL-6 Antibodies

As mentioned above, IL-6 is a crucial pro-inflammatory cytokine in infection and tissue injury [16]. It initiates the differentiation of immune cells and early inflammatory reactions. Study has shown that the serum level of IL-6 was related to severe COVID-19 and indicated a worse prognosis, including ICU admission, respiratory failure, and even death. The IL-6 in COVID-19 patients is a symbol of CRS [17]. This part would introduce a few anti-IL-6 antibodies; some are already approved for autoimmune disease, and others are in the experimental stage.

Tocilizumab is an anti-IL6 receptor humanized monoclonal antibody used in rheumatologic disease with good efficacy. Moreover, it was approved by the FDA for the treatment of CRS. One meta-analysis indicates that tocilizumab could reduce mortality and other relevant outcomes in hospitalized patients [18]. Evidence supports that tocilizumab positively affects severe COVID-19 patients. Using tocilizumab significantly decreases IL-6 level and C reaction protein, indicating relief in a cytokine storm [19]. Although tocilizumab did have a good outcome for severe patients, some studies revealed different conclusions. One meta-analysis suggested that tocilizumab had no effect on short-term mortality (the first month). However, the tocilizumab did reduce the mechanical ventilation rate and improve the blood oxygen level [20]. However, some random clinical trials (RCT) showed conflicting results. Three RCTs conducted a method that involved patients randomly, double-blind in a 2:1 ratio to receive standard care plus a single dose of tocilizumab (8 mg/kg) or placebo. All results suggested that tocilizumab was inadequate to improve survival or clinical situation in 28 days. However, the tocilizumab reduced the possibilities of the composite outcome of mechanical ventilation or death [21, 22, 23]. These conflicting results may indicate that the inflammatory pathways involved in COVID-19 are very complicated. Only conducting single-target medicine won't improve patients' survival or general clinical situations.

Sarilumab is a humanized monoclonal antibody that targets the IL-6 receptor, like tocilizumab. One review supports sarilumab is a safe medicine with good efficacy in COVID-19 patients, and can be an alternative treatment option [24, 25]. One meta-analysis collected 27 RCTs of 13 549 patients receiving corticosteroid treatment, to confirm whether sarilumab and baricitinib were non-inferior to tocilizumab. Results showed that sarilumab and baricitinib had a similar effect on reducing mortality and they have no difference with tocilizumab. That provides an alternative to baricitinib in cases where it is not available, such as gastrointestinal absorption dysfunction, renal failure, or pregnant patients [26]. Like tocilizumab, several random clinical trials don't observe improvement in the sarilumab group compared to placebo [27, 28]. While there are still encouraging results. One RCT evaluated the difference between sarilumab, tocilizumab, and standard care, sorting 353 patients in the ICU. Results showed that the sarilumab and tocilizumab group improved outcomes and survival [29]. Interestingly, combining sarilumab or tocilizumab with corticosteroids may have a better effect on patients than on corticosteroids alone. One meta-analysis revealed that the patients with severe COVID-19 in hospitals who received sarilumab and corticosteroids had lower mortality than the single corticosteroids group. When used tocilizumab and corticosteroids as treatment, they have a similar effect compared with sarilumab and corticosteroids. However, using sarilumab or tocilizumab alone didn't improve significantly [30].

Siltuximab is an anti-IL-6 antibody. It's a chimeric human-mouse monoclonal antibody that is used for Castleman disease. One study suggested that siltuximab could be considered a therapeutic medicine for COVID-19, as it blocked both soluble and membrane-bound IL-6. The efficacy of siltuximab cannot be valued by the IL-6 in blood because the siltuximab-IL-6 complex interferes with the detection of IL-6. It recommended suppressing C reactive protein as the measurement method [31]. As for the comparison between siltuximab and tocilizumab, one study demonstrated that siltuximab was a well-tolerated alternative medicine to tocilizumab. It concluded that 31 patients with comorbidities such as hypertension, chronic respiratory disease, cardiomyopathy, and a median age of 62. Some patients received siltuximab or tocilizumab alone; some received tocilizumab and then turned to siltuximab. The patients who were treated with siltuximab or tocilizumab alone had a similar mortality. But on the other hand, replacing tocilizumab with siltuximab didn't show a better efficacy. This group even had a worse outcome [32]. The reason might be that these 2 antibodies have the exact mechanism; if the patients didn't respond to tocilizumab, their pathogenic mechanisms were probably not the IL-6 pathway.

ALD518 is an antibody that targets IL-6, developed to treat lung cancer. Although its original function is not aimed at infectious disease, the typical inflammatory pathway of cytokine storm and lung cancer makes it a new medicine to CRS [33]. ADL518 is still in the experimental stage; no clinical data confirms its role in treatment. Whether it could be another antibody to cure COVID-19 needs more data support.

Anti-IFN-γ Antibodies

IFN-γ is a cytokine involved in several inflammatory pathways and immune cells, including NK cells, macrophages, and T cells, and connects natural immune and adaptive immune. IFN-γ is a significant factor in hemophagocytic lymphohistiocytosis (HLH), an excessive immune reaction that damages the tissue with clinical symptoms [2]. Thus, IFN-γ is an indication of the cytokine storm.

Emapalumab is an anti-IFN-γ monoclonal antibody approved by the FDA in 2018 to treat HLH [34]. There is a study that described the clinical efficacy of emapalumab in curing HLH caused by EBV. This study also mentioned that IFN-γ would lead to immune system overreacts [35]. Meanwhile, some studies indicate that type Ⅰ and Ⅲ IFNs play essential roles in the infection of SARS-CoV-2[36]. However, a study pointed out that the mechanism of CRS caused by COVID-19 was different from HLH because they were both overactive inflammatory reactions. COVID-19 patients have low levels of Fas ligand, while HLH patients have an activation of the IL-18-IFN-γ axis [37]. Besides, the clinical evidence of the efficacy of emapalumab for COVID-19 is insufficient. No RCT has been conducted to evaluate the safety and effect of emapalumab when used in COVID-19. Thus, we need more research to confirm the role of emapalumab in treating COVID-19.

Discussion

Many clinical doctors conduct glucocorticoids to cure cytokine storms, widely used in COVID-19. Compared to glucocorticoids, the anti-inflammatory antibodies have both advantages and disadvantages. Large amounts of glucocorticoids would cause side effects, including Cushing's syndrome, water-sodium metabolism disorder, osteolysis, and immunosuppression. However, the anti-inflammatory antibodies could aim at only the inflammatory pathway with no metabolic side effects. Antibodies can only target one particular inflammatory factor or one pathway, while glucocorticoids effectively inhibit multiple inflammatory pathways and productions. This might be a plus or minus for anti-inflammatory antibodies. As mentioned above, there are conflicting results in RCTs of tocilizumab. The pathways of cytokine storm caused by infectious disease may differ from rheumatic diseases, which means the multiple mechanisms behind the infectious disease that the single target treatment strategy cannot work. The transportation and preservation of antibodies are more stringent than chemicals, making them natural disadvantages. This will raise the cost of antibodies and lead to less consideration of antibodies. Also, some cytokine inhibitors are not antibodies, such as anakinra and etanercept. Anakinra is a recombinant IL-1 receptor antagonist for blocking the IL-1 signal. Many studies and trials have revealed the positive effect of anakinra on COVID-19 patients, including reducing mortality, decreasing the inflammatory level, shortening hospitalization, and protecting patients from respiratory failure [38, 39]. The anakinra is not omnipotent, the administration time and treatment type are essential factors to the outcome of anakinra. The earlier anakinra is used, the better prognosis patients will have. For those who already have respiratory failure, anakinra may not show improvements [40]. More evidence is needed to confirm whether canakinumab or other factor antibodies have a better effect.

The anti-inflammatory antibody is an option for sever COVID-19 but not the only solution. Besides medical measures, blood purification is complementary to curing cytokine storms [41]. Although we have so many measures to combat systemic inflammatory reactions or cytokine storms, the mortality of COVID-19 doesn't lie; the severe COVID-19 did take many lives. Because the mechanisms behind the cytokine storm caused by infection are still unclear. The effect of aiming for one cytokine may be limited. Treatment targets multiple cytokines or pathways in the clinic, such as bispecific antibodies aiming at two inflammatory factors, are needed, including medicine measures or invasive measures. Besides, anti-inflammatory antibodies need more RCT evidence to support that this treatment has more effect and fewer side effects than traditional measures.

References

[1] Xiaobo Yang, Yuan Yu, Jiqian Xu, Huaqing Shu, Jia'an Xia, Hong Liu, Yongran Wu, Lu Zhang, Zhui Yu, Minghao Fang, Ting Yu, Yaxin Wang, Shangwen Pan, Xiaojing Zou, Shiying Yuan, You Shang. 2020. Clinical course and outcomes of critically ill patients with SARS-CoV-2 pneumonia in Wuhan, China: a single-centered, retrospective, observational study. *Lancet Respir Med.* 8(5):475-481.

[2] Jae Seok Kim, Jun Young Lee, Jae Won Yang, Keum Hwa Lee, Maria Effenberger, Wladimir Szpirt, Andreas Kronbichler, Jae Il Shin. 2021. Immunopathogenesis and treatment of cytokine storm in COVID-19. *Theranostics*, 11(1):316-329.

[3] Konstantin Doberer, Michael Duerr, Philip F. Halloran, Farsad Eskandary, Klemens Budde, Heinz Regele, Jeff Reeve, Anita Borski, Nicolas Kozakowski, Roman Reindl-Schwaighofer, Johannes Waiser, Nils Lachmann, Sabine Schranz, Christa Firbas, Jakob Mühlbacher, Georg Gelbenegger, Thomas Perkmann, Markus Wahrmann, Alexander Kainz, Robin Ristl, Fabian Halleck, Gregor Bond, Edward Chong, Bernd Jilma, Georg A. Böhmig. 2021. A Randomized Clinical Trial of Anti-IL-6 Antibody Clazakizumab in Late Antibody-Mediated Kidney Transplant Rejection. *J Am Soc Nephrol,* 32(3): 708-722.

[4] Eric A Coomes, Hourmazd Haghbayan. 2020. Interleukin-6 in Covid-19: A systematic review and meta-analysis. *Rev Med Virol*, 30(6): 1-9.

[5] Dennis McGonagle, Kassem Sharif, Anthony O'Regan, Charlie Bridgewood. 2020. The Role of Cytokines including Interleukin-6 in COVID-19 induced Pneumonia and Macrophage Activation Syndrome-Like Disease. *Autoimmun Rev*, 19(6): 102537.

[6] Nora Müller, Jens van den Brandt, Francesca Odoardi, Denise Tischner, Judith Herath, Alexander Flügel, Holger M Reichardt. 2008. A CD28 superagonistic antibody elicits 2 functionally distinct waves of T cell activation in rats. *J Clin Invest*, 118(4):1405-1416.

[7] Ruan Q, Yang K, Wang W, Jiang L, Song J. 2020. Clinical predictors of mortality due to COVID-19 based on an analysis of data of 150 patients from Wuhan, China. *Intensive Care Med.* 46(5):846-848.

[8] Miriam Merad, Catherine A. Blish, Federica Sallusto, Aikio Iwasaki. 2022. The immunology and immunopathology of COVID-19. *Nature*, 375(6585):1122-1127.

[9] Christoph Schultheiß, Edith Willscher, Lisa Paschold, Cornelia Gottschick, Bianca Klee, Svenja-Sibylla Henkes, Lidia Bosurgi, Jochen Dutzmann 4 Daniel Sedding, Thomas Frese, Matthias Girndt, Jessica I Höll, Michael Gekle, Rafael Mikolajczyk, Mascha Binder. 2022. The IL-1β, IL-6, and TNF cytokine triad is associated with post-acute sequelae of COVID-19. *Cell Rep Med*, 21;3(6):100663.

[10] Leigh D Church, Michael F McDermott. 2010. Canakinumab: a human anti-IL-1β monoclonal antibody for the treatment of cryopyrin-associated periodic syndromes. *Expert Rev Clin Immunol*, 6(6): 831-841.

[11] Eugen Dhimolea. 2010. Canakinumab. *Mabs*, 2(1): 3-13.

[12] Frank L. van de Veerdonk, Mihai G. Netea. 2020. Blocking IL-1 to prevent respiratory failure in COVID-19. *Crit Care*, 24: 4445.

[13] Guangyu Ao, Yushu Wang, Anthony Li, Carolyn Tran, D, Qing Yang. 2020. The effect of canakinumab on clinical outcomes in patients with COVID-19: A meta-analysis. *J Infect*, 84(6): 834-872.

[14] Daniele Generali, Giancarlo Bosio, Fabio Malberti, Antonio Cuzzoli, Sophie Testa, Laura Romanini, Antonio Fioravanti, Alessandro Morandini, Luca Pianta, Guglielmo Giannotti, Erika Maria Viola, Matteo Giorgi-Pierfranceschi, Marina Foramitti, Rosa Angela Tira, Ilaria Zangrandi, Giulia Chiodelli, Andrea Machiavelli, Maria Rosa Cappelletti, Alessia Giossi, Valeria De Giuli, Chiara Costanzi, Chiara Campana, Ottavia Bernocchi, Marianna Sirico, Alessia Zoncada, Alfredo Molteni, Sergio Venturini, Fabiola Giudici, Maurizio Scaltriti, Angelo Pan. 2021. Canakinumab as treatment for COVID-19-related pneumonia: A prospective case-control study. *Int J Infect Dis*, 104: 433-440.

[15] Matthias Hepprich, Jonathan M Mudry, Claudia Gregoriano, Francois R Jornayvaz, Sebastian Carballo, Anne Wojtusciszynm, Pierre-Alexandre Bart, Jean-Daniel Chiche, Stefan Fischli, Thomas Baumgartner, Claudia Cavelti-Weder, Dominique L Braun, Huldrych F Günthard, Felix Beuschlein, Anna Conen, Emily West, Egon Isenring, Stefan Zechmann, Gabriela Bucklar, Yoann Aubry, Ludovic Dey, Beat Müller, Patrick Hunziker, Philipp Schütz, Marco Cattaneo, Marc Y Donath. 2022. Canakinumab in patients with COVID-19 and type 2 diabetes - A multicentre, randomised, double-blind, placebo-controlled trial. *EClinicalMedicine*, 53:101649.

[16] Toshio Tanaka, Masashi Narazaki, Tadamitsu Kishimoto. 2014. IL-6 in inflammation, immunity, and disease. *Cold Spring Harb Perspect Biol*, 6(10): a016295.

[17] Eric A Coomes, Hourmazd Haghbayan. 2020. Interleukin-6 in Covid-19: A systematic review and meta-analysis. *Rev Med Virol*, 30(6):1-9.

[18] Christos Kyriakopoulos, Georgios Ntritsos, Athena Gogali, Haralampos Milionis, Evangelos Evangelou, Konstantinos Kostikas. 2021. Tocilizumab administration for the treatment of hospitalized patients with COVID-19: A systematic review and meta-analysis. *Respirology,* 26(11): 1027-1040.

[19] Christos Kyriakopoulos, Georgios Ntritsos, Athena Gogali, Haralampos Milionis, Evangelos Evangelou, Konstantinos Kostikas. 2021. Tocilizumab administration for the treatment of hospitalized patients with COVID-19: A systematic review and meta-analysis. *Respirology*, 26(11): 1027-1040.

[20] Timothée Klopfenstein, Vincent Gendrin, N'dri Juliette Kadiane-Oussou, Thierry Conrozier, Souheil Zayet. 2022. Tocilizumab in COVID-19 pneumonia: Practical proposals based on a narrative review of randomised trials. *Rev Med Virol*, 32(1): e2239.

[21] John H. Stone, Matthew J. Frigault, Naomi J. Serling-Boyd, Ana D. Fernandes., Liam Harvey, Andrea S. Foulkes, Nora K. Horick, Brian C. Healy, Ruta Shah, Ana

Maria Bensaci, Ann E. Woolley, Sarah Nikiforow, Nina Lin, Manish Sagar, Harry Schrager, David S. Huckins, Matthew Axelrod, Michael D. Pincus, Jorge Fleisher, Chana A. Sacks, Michael Dougan, Crystal M. North, Yuan-Di Halvorsen, Tara K. Thurber, Zeina Dagher, Allison Scherer, Rachel S. Wallwork, Arthur Y. Kim, Sara Schoenfeld, Pritha Sen, Tomas G. Neilan, Cory A. Perugino, Sebastian H. Unizony, Deborah S. Collier, Mark A. Matza, Janeth M. Yinh, Kathryn A. Bowman, Eric Meyerowitz, Amna Zafar, Zsofia D. Drobni, Marcy B. Bolster, Minna Kohler, Kristin M. D'Silva., Jonathan Dau, Megan M. Lockwood, Caroline Cubbison, Brittany N. Weber, Michael K. Mansour. 2020. Efficacy of Tocilizumab in Patients Hospitalized with Covid-19. *N Engl J Med*, 383:2333-2344.

[22] Carlos Salama, Jian Han, Linda Yau, William G. Reiss, Benjamin Kramer, Jeffrey D. Neidhart, Gerard J. Criner, Emma Kaplan-Lewis, Rachel Baden, Lavannya Pandit, Miriam L. Cameron, Julia Garcia-Diaz, Victoria Chávez, Martha Mekebeb-Reuter, Ferdinando Lima de Menezes, Reena Shah, Maria F. González-Lara, Beverly Assman, Jamie Freedman, Shalini V. Mohan. 2021. Tocilizumab in Patients Hospitalized with Covid-19 Pneumonia. *N Engl J Med*, 384:20-30.

[23] Ivan O. Rosas, Norbert Bräu, Michael Waters, Ronaldo C. Go, Bradley D. Hunter, Sanjay Bhagani, Daniel Skiest, Mariam S. Aziz, Nichola Cooper, Ivor S. Douglas, Sinisa Savic, Taryn Youngstein, Lorenzo Del Sorbo, Antonio Cubillo Gracian, David J. De La Zerda, Andrew Ustianowski, Min Bao, Sophie Dimonaco, Emily Graham, Balpreet Matharu, Helen Spotswood, Larry Tsai, Atul Malhotra. 2021. Tocilizumab in Hospitalized Patients with Severe Covid-19 Pneumonia. *N Engl J Med*, 384:1503-1516.

[24] Bingwen Liu, Min Li, Zhiguang Zhou, Xuan Guan, Yufei Xiang. 2020. Can we use interleukin-6 (IL-6) blockade for coronavirus disease 2019 (COVID-19)-induced cytokine release syndrome (CRS)? *J Autoimmun*, 111:102452.

[25] Andrea Marino, Antonio Munafò, Egle Augello, Carlo Maria Bellanca, Carmelo Bonomo, Manuela Ceccarelli, Nicolò Musso, Giuseppina Cantarella, Bruno Cacopardo, Renato Bernardini. 2022. Sarilumab Administration in COVID-19 Patients: Literature Review and Considerations. *Infect Dis Rep,* 14(3):360-371.

[26] Arthur M. Albuquerque, Igor Eckert, Lucas Tramujas, Guillaume Butler-Laporte, Emily G. McDonald, James M. Brophy, Todd C. Lee. 2023. Effect of tocilizumab, sarilumab, and baricitinib on mortality among patients hospitalized for COVID-19 treated with corticosteroids: a systematic review and meta-analysis. *Clin Microbiol Infect*, 29(1): 13–21.

[27] François-Xavier Lescure, Hitoshi Honda, Robert A Fowler, Jennifer Sloane Lazar, Genming Shi, Peter Wung, Naimish Patel, Owen Hagino. 2021. Sarilumab in patients admitted to hospital with severe or critical COVID-19: a randomised, double-blind, placebo-controlled, phase 3 trial. *Lancet Respir Med*, 9(5): 522–532.

[28] The CORIMUNO-19 Collaborative group. 2022. Sarilumab in adults hospitalised with moderate-to-severe COVID-19 pneumonia (CORIMUNO-SARI-1): An open-label randomised controlled trial. *Lancet Rheumatol*, 4(1): e24–e32.

[29] Anthony C Gordon, Paul R Mouncey, Farah Al-Beidh, Kathryn M Rowan, Alistair D Nichol, Yaseen M Arabi, Djillali Annane, Abi Beane, Wilma van Bentum-Puijk, Lindsay R Berry, Zahra Bhimani, Marc J M Bonten, Charlotte A Bradbury, Frank

M Brunkhorst, Adrian Buzgau, Allen C Cheng, Michelle A Detry, Eamon J Duffy, Lise J Estcourt, Mark Fitzgerald, Herman Goossens, Rashan Haniffa, Alisa M Higgins, Thomas E Hills, Christopher M Horvat, Francois Lamontagne, Patrick R Lawler, Helen L Leavis, Kelsey M Linstrum, Edward Litton, Elizabeth Lorenzi, John C Marshall, Florian B Mayr, Daniel F McAuley, Anna McGlothlin, Shay P McGuinness, Bryan J McVerry, Stephanie K Montgomery, Susan C Morpeth, Srinivas Murthy, Katrina Orr, Rachael L Parke, Jane C Parker, Asad E Patanwala, Ville Pettilä, Emma Rademaker, Marlene S Santos, Christina T Saunders, Christopher W Seymour, Manu Shankar-Hari, Wendy I Sligl, Alexis F Turgeon, Anne M Turner, Frank L van de Veerdonk, Ryan Zarychanski, Cameron Green, Roger J Lewis, Derek C Angus, Colin J McArthur, Scott Berry, Steve A Webb, Lennie P G Derde. 2021. Interleukin-6 Receptor Antagonists in Critically Ill Patients with Covid-19. *N Engl J Med*, 384(16):1491-1502.

[30] Dena Zeraatkar, Ellen Cusano, Juan Pablo Díaz Martínez, Anila Qasim, Sophia Mangala, Elena Kum, Jessica Julia Bartoszko, Tahira Devji, Thomas Agoritsas, Gordon Guyatt, Ariel Izcovich, Assem M Khamis, Francois Lamontagne, Bram Rochwerg, Per Vandvik, Romina Brignardello-Petersen, Reed Alexander Cunningham Siemieniuk. 2022. Use of tocilizumab and sarilumab alone or in combination with corticosteroids for covid-19: systematic review and network meta-analysis. *BMJ Med*, 28;1(1): e000036.

[31] Tomás Palanques-Pastor, Eduardo López-Briz, José Luis Poveda Andrés. 2020. Involvement of interleukin 6 in SARS-CoV-2 infection: siltuximab as a therapeutic option against COVID-19. *Eur J Hosp Pharm*, 27(5): 297–298.

[32] Fernanda Meira, Laia Albiach, Cristina Carbonell, José-Ángel Martín-Oterino, Mercedes Martín-Ordiales, Laura Linares, Irene Macaya, Daiana Agüero, Juan Ambrosioni, Marta Bodro, Celia Cardozo, Mariana Chumbita, Lorena De la Mora, Nicole García-Pouton, Carolina Garcia-Vidal, Ana González-Cordón, Marta Hernández-Meneses, Alexy Inciarte, Montserrat Laguno, Lorna Leal, Laura Morata, Pedro Puerta-Alcalde, Verónica Rico, Laura Letona, Alberto Cózar-Llistó, Gerard Dueñas, Montserrat Solá, Berta Torres, Jhon Rojas, Antonio Moreno, Estela Moreno-García, Manuel Torres, José A Martínez, Alex Soriano, Felipe García. 2021. Experience with the use of siltuximab in patients with SARS-CoV-2 infection. *Rev Esp Quimioter*, 34(4): 337–341.

[33] Trevor J Bayliss, Jeff T Smith, Michael Schuster, Konstantin H Dragnev, James R Rigas, 2011, A humanized anti-IL-6 antibody (ALD518) in non-small cell lung cancer. *Expert Opin Biol Ther*, 11(12):1663-1668.

[34] Mounica Vallurupalli, Nancy Berliner. 2019. Emapalumab for the treatment of relapsed/refractory hemophagocytic lymphohistiocytosis. *Blood*, 134(21): 1783-1786.

[35] Dana T Lounder, Qiong Bin, Cristina de Min, Michael B Jordan. 2019. Treatment of refractory hemophagocytic lymphohistiocytosis with emapalumab despite severe concurrent infections. *Blood Adv*, 3(1):47-50.

[36] Dhiraj Acharya, GuanQun Liu, Michaela U Gack. 2020. Dysregulation of type I interferon responses in COVID-19. *Nat Rev Immunol,* 20(7): 397-398.

[37] Johnson M Liu, Jeffrey Chi. 2022. Is COVID-19-associated cytokine storm distinct from non-COVID-19 secondary hemophagocytic lymphohistiocytosis? *Exp Biol Med (Maywood)*. 247(4): 330–337.

[38] A García-Lledó, J Gómez-Pavón, J González Del Castillo, T Hernández-Sampelayo, M C Martín-Delgado, F J Martín Sánchez, M Martínez-Sellés, J M Molero García, S Moreno Guillén, F J Rodríguez-Artalejo, J Ruiz-Galiana, R Cantón, P De Lucas Ramos, A García-Botella, E Bouza. 2021. Pharmacological treatment of COVID-19: an opinion paper. *Rev Esp Quimioter*, 35(2): 115-130.

[39] Evdoxia Kyriazopoulou, Thomas Huet, Giulio Cavalli, Andrea Gori, Miltiades Kyprianou, Peter Pickkers, Jesper Eugen-Olsen, Mario Clerici, Francisco Veas, Gilles Chatellier, Gilles Kaplanski, Mihai G Netea, Emanuele Pontali, Marco Gattorno, Raphael Cauchois, Emma Kooistra, Matthijs Kox, Alessandra Bandera, Hélène Beaussier, Davide Mangioni, Lorenzo Dagna, Jos W M van der Meer, Evangelos J Giamarellos-Bourboulis, Gilles Hayem. 2021. Effect of anakinra on mortality in patients with COVID-19: a systematic review and patient-level meta-analysis. *Lancet Rheumatol*, 3(10): e690-e697.

[40] Elnaz Khani, Marzieh Shahrabi, Haleh Rezaei, Fariba Pourkarim, Hoda Afsharirad, Mohammad Solduzian. 2022. Current evidence on the use of anakinra in COVID-19. *Int Immunopharmacol*. 111: 109075.

[41] Shi-Long Yang, Xiao-Jun Xu, Yong-Min Tang, Hua Song, Wei-Qun Xu, Fen-Ying Zhao, Di-Ying Shen. 2016. Associations between inflammatory cytokines and organ damage in pediatric patients with hemophagocytic lymphohistiocytosis. *Cytokine,* 85:14-7.

Biographical Sketch

Jiayang Wang

Affiliation: BSL-3 Laboratory (Guangdong), Guangdong Provincial Key Laboratory of Tropical Disease Research, School of Public Health, Southern Medical University, Guangzhou, People's Republic of China.

Education: 2017-2022 Graduated from the Southern Medical University major in Traditional Chinese Medicine and Western Medicine in Clinical.

Business Address: 1023-1063 Shatai Nan Road, Guangzhou, Guangdong Province, China.

Chapter 9

Nanobodies in Human Infectious Diseases: A Comprehensive Review of Research and Applications

Ziyou Chen[1,2,4]
Yuanzhi Chen[1,2,4,†]
Zhiren Zeng[1,2,4]
Na Yuan[1,2]
Yaxian Mei[1,3]
Zhenzhen Zhu[1,2]
and Wenxin Luo[1,2,†]

[1]State Key Laboratory of Molecular Vaccinology and Molecular Diagnostics; National Institute of Diagnostics and Vaccine, Development in Infectious Diseases, School of Public Health, School of Life Sciences, Xiamen University, Xiamen, China

[2]Xiang An Biomedicine Laboratory, Xiamen, China

[3]Brand Innovation Department, Hangzhou Innovax Biotech Co. Ltd, Hangzhou, Zhejiang, China

[4]These authors contributed equally to this work.

Abstract

Infectious diseases, triggered by pathogenic microorganisms, have the potential to lead to global crises. Beyond enduring infectious illnesses such as malaria and dengue fever, recent malevolent outbreaks of diseases like Neocon, Ebola, SARS-CoV, MERS-CoV, and SARS-CoV-

[†]Corresponding Author's E-mail: chenyuanzhi939@gmail.com
[†]Corresponding Author's E-mail: wxluo@xmu.edu.cn.

In: Neutralizing Antibodies and their Role in Health and Disease
Editors: Chenguang Shen, Yang Yang and Minghui Yang
ISBN: 979-8-89113-541-3

2 have accelerated the search for more effective and accessible methods for improved diagnosis and treatment. Among the various avenues explored, antibodies have gained significant attention owing to their favorable structural characteristics and versatile applications. Nanobodies, also referred to as single domain-based VHHs and derived from heavy-chain only IgG antibodies found in the Camillidae family, can stably bind to antigens and offer a host of advantages such as high stability, pronounced hydrophilicity, and ease of expression and modification. These attributes allow them to directly target antigen epitopes or be engineered into multivalent nanobodies or nanobody fusion proteins to wield therapeutic effects. This paper provides an in-depth examination of the methods used to construct nanobodies and explores their potential functions, summarizing the current progress of research in the field and underscoring their diverse applications in the management and understanding of human infectious diseases.

Introduction

Microorganisms serve a crucial role in our ecosystem, yet certain microbes such as viruses, bacteria, fungi, and their toxic products can become pathogenic, exerting a substantial burden on global healthcare. The World Health Organization has reported millions of deaths attributed to communicable diseases in the past year alone. According to a survey by the World Health Organization, millions succumbed to communicable diseases in just a single year. While we grapple with enduring communicable diseases such as malaria, dengue, human immunodeficiency virus (HIV), Human papillomavirus (HPV), and Hepatitis B virus (HBV), we are also confronted by outbreaks such as the Spanish Flu, Ebola, Zika, SARS-CoV, MERS-CoV, and notably, SARS-CoV-2. It's worth highlighting that the novel coronavirus (SARS-CoV-2), has accounted for more than 7.6 million deaths globally as of August 1st, 2023 (WHO coronavirus (COVID-19) dashboard: https://covid19.who.int/). Such alarming statistics necessitate the exploration of novel diagnostic and treatment strategies beyond existing antimicrobial drugs. The technological advancements in recent years have facilitated the development of innovative tools in scientific research, opening new therapeutic avenues. A prominent development in this domain is the rise of antibody-based immunotherapy. Antibodies (Abs) have become an appealing biomolecule for diagnosing and treating infectious diseases due to their target specificity, structural flexibility, and diversity. Among the various antibody-based molecules, nanobodies (Nbs) have emerged as suitable candidates for both diagnostics and therapeutics in the fight against infectious diseases. These natural small molecule antibodies are garnering attention for their increasing role in the treatment of such diseases. Currently, several nanobodies are undergoing clinical testing, including MucoRice-ARP1 for rotavirus [1, 2] and ALX-0171 for respiratory syncytial virus (RSV). During the COVID-19 pandemic, numerous nanobodies targeting SARS-CoV-2 have been identified and engineered into different forms, such as bivalent, bispecific, and trivalent structures, exhibiting promising therapeutic effects in ex vivo and in vivo experiments. In this study, we elucidate the construction methods and potential functions of nanobodies, summarizing their recent advances in the realm of infectious diseases. By weaving together a comprehensive understanding of nanobodies and their applications, we hope to contribute valuable insights that may guide future research and intervention strategies in the ongoing battle against global infectious diseases.

Characteristics of Nanobody

Nanobodies were first identified in camelids by Hamers-Casterman and his team in 1993. They discovered the presence of heavy-chain-only antibodies (HCAbs) in camelids, comprising a CH2 constant domain, a CH3 constant domain, a hinge region, and a variable heavy chain domain (VHH), with the latter also referred to as a nanobody [3]. Distinct from the conventional antibody with a molecular weight of 150 kDa and fragments like Fabs (50 kDa) and scFv (25 kDa), nanobodies are markedly smaller, weighing in at only 15 kDa [4]. As the smallest known single-domain antibodies, nanobodies lack a light chain, which simplifies their post-translational modifications and facilitates diverse expression systems. Structurally, nanobodies consist of four framework regions (FR1, FR2, FR3, FR4) and three complementarity-determining regions (CDR1, CDR2, CDR3). The CDR3 region, which plays a vital role in antigen binding in nanobodies, tends to be longer and exhibits increased amino acid residue variability compared to conventional Abs. As a result, nanobodies can bind with high affinity and recognize a broader spectrum of epitopes, including some 'hidden' or cryptic ones [5-7]. Additionally, unique structural features, such as four hydrophilic amino acid residues in FR2 and a disulfide bond between CDR1 and CDR3, endow them with high solubility and stability under extreme pH or temperature conditions. These characteristics prove beneficial for drug preservation and delivery, facilitating oral or nasal drug uptake routes [8-10]. While the immunogenicity of antibodies can induce serious in vivo side effects, especially at high doses, humanization processes can mitigate these concerns. Humanizing antibodies effectively reduces their immunogenicity while retaining specificity and affinity, enhancing their therapeutic applicability [11]. Nanobodies exhibit a natural advantage in this regard, as they show high homology with human VH domains, which simplifies human source transformation and minimizes clinical side effects. Traditional humanization of VHH involves the replacement of framework residues with corresponding residues of human VH, avoiding specific substitutions in hydrophilic amino acids [12]. Further, nanobodies can be humanized through straightforward site-directed mutagenesis, given the compact gene size of approximately 380 bp [4, 13]. Researchers such as Vincke and colleagues have humanized VHH by substituting 12 amino acid residues differing from the corresponding region of human VH [13]. In sum, the distinct advantages of nanobodies, encompassing their size, structure, binding characteristics, and ease of humanization, render them highly promising tools in the battle against infectious diseases. Their potential for targeted therapy and diagnostic applications continues to stimulate innovative research and development, positioning them at the forefront of infectious disease intervention strategies.

Construction of Nanobody Library

Antigen-specific nanobodies are predominantly sourced from constructed libraries, which can be categorized into immune, naïve, or synthetic VHH libraries [14]. Among these, immune libraries are often considered the most efficient avenue for obtaining functional nanobodies. As depicted in Figure 1, the construction of immune libraries commences with the active immunization of Camillidae animals, such as dromedaries, alpacas, llamas, and heavy chain only antibodies (HCAbs) transgenic mice, using specific immunogens [15, 16]. These immunogens stimulate the immune system to produce HCAbs that exhibit reasonable specificity and high affinity [12]. Subsequently, lymphocytes are isolated from the host for mRNA extraction, followed by reverse transcription to obtain cDNA fragments. VHH sequences are then amplified through nested Polymerase Chain Reactions (PCRs), and the distinct sequences are inserted into vectors for transformation into an expression system. A nanobody (Nb) library with more than 10^7 individual transformants is deemed of adequate quality for subsequent screening [17]. Naïve libraries offer more convenience, relying on the inherent immunological diversity within camelids without necessitating active immunization. They also enable the identification of nanobodies binding to specific antigens, such as non-immunogenic or toxic ones [18]. However, their size and diversity limitations impede efficient screening. Naïve libraries typically require 10^9–10^{10} individual clones, obtained from large blood samples (> 10 L) across different animals to mitigate bias [17]. Synthetic libraries, constructed through targeted mutagenesis in specialized CDR regions, provide sufficiently diverse options for nanobody screening [14, 19]. Like naïve libraries, they permit screening without immunization but necessitate a more intricate and effective design, along with a larger library size ranging from 10^9 to 10^15 to find targeting nanobodies [17]. A systematic approach to constructing synthetic libraries encompasses the selection of proper framework sequences, the randomization of CDRs, and the synthesis of diverse DNA sequences. Optimization of factors like primer quality, DNA polymerase fidelity, and experimental techniques can control undesirable frameshift mutations, enhancing the quality of synthetic libraries [16]. Despite these methods, obtaining suitable nanobodies can prove challenging due to the extensive diversity of libraries or other inherent limitations. In such scenarios, selected nanobodies may be enhanced in affinity through molecular techniques, such as error-prone PCR, DNA family shuffling, and site-specific amino acid mutations [6, 20, 21]. These refinement methods further expand the potential applications of nanobodies, underscoring their emerging role as versatile tools in diagnostic and therapeutic strategies for infectious diseases.

Production Systems for Nanobodies

Nanobodies are produced through two primary expression systems: prokaryotic and eukaryotic (Figure 1). The bacterial expression systems, especially those utilizing E. coli, are the most commonly chosen methods due to their ease of purification and low cost [22]. Additionally, yeast and fungal expression systems have proven suitable for high nanobody production [6, 23, 24]. Mammalian cells such as HEK293T cells, CHO cells, and Expi293F are favorable choices for producing various forms of nanobodies, including VHH-Fc fusions and Nbs-HRP fusions [6, 25]. Ario provided further examples of mammalian cell expression [25]. When nanobodies (Nbs) are fused with tags to facilitate purification, bacterial expression can also be employed [26, 27]. The expression systems determine the approach to nanobody screening. E. coli-based phage display technique is widely used, where Fv genes are displayed on the phage surface alongside phage coat proteins [16]. Phages secreted by E. coli can bind to targeted antigens on solid surfaces, followed by amplification and consecutive screening to identify suitable antigen-specific phages. This process, although effective, may be time-consuming. In vitro assays like phage ELISA help identify phages displaying nanobodies with the desired affinity [14, 28]. Additionally, platforms such as yeast surface display have been constructed for specific applications, like targeting human G-protein-coupled receptors [29], or screening nanobodies against the Receptor Binding Domain (RBD) of SARS-CoV-2 [30]. Diverse expression systems have expanded the application of nanobodies, particularly in combating gastrointestinal and genital tract diseases. Nanobodies can maintain functionality under extreme conditions, resisting pepsin, and performing well in both digestive and genital tracts. This property enables patients to consume foods like Arabidopsis thaliana seeds and rice expressing nanobodies as a protective measure. An innovative example is MucoRice-ARP1, a transgenic rice expressing anti-rotavirus nanobodies [1]. Currently in clinical trials, this rice-based solution is promising as an oral, mass-producible anti-rotavirus product, maintaining activity even after boiling and demonstrating efficacy in animal experiments. In the realm of gastrointestinal mucosa protection, seed-bioencapsulated SIgA-analog (sVHH-IgA) has been produced in Arabidopsis by replacing the antigen-binding fragment of IgA with a nanobody [31, 32]. Such developments have led to reduced bacterial shedding and immunity response in piglets. Similarly, fused chimeric antibodies targeting Campylobacter have been efficiently expressed in plants like Nicotiana benthamiana and Arabidopsis thaliana, contributing to passive oral immunization in chickens [33]. Nanobodies also bring forth new strategies for preventing sexually transmitted diseases (STDs), such as AIDS. An exciting development is the expression of the HIV-neutralizing nanobody VHH A6 in Lactobacillus rhamnosus DSM 14870, a strain that can colonize the human vagina [34]. This approach is expected to be used for high-risk HIV women and represents an innovative and economic supplement to current vaccine-based prevention strategies

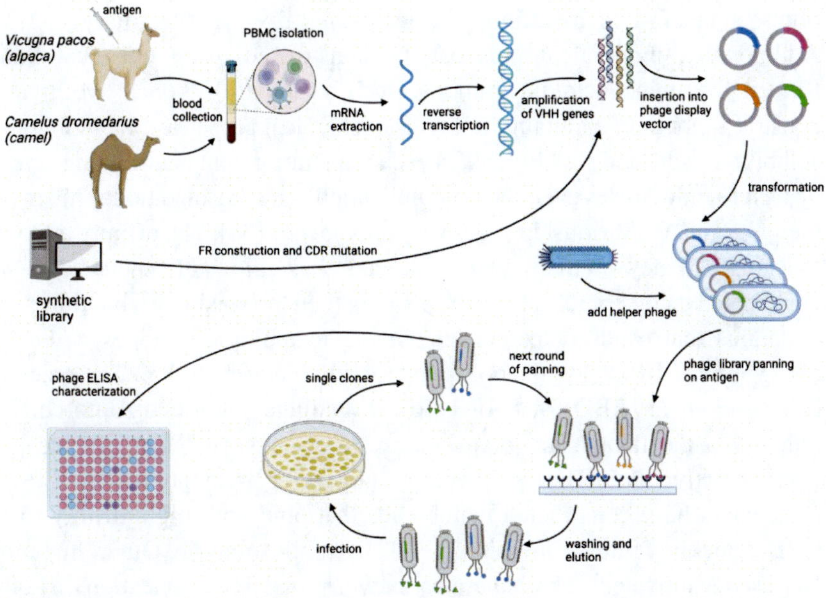

Figure 1. Illustrative overview of nanobody production utilizing both phage display libraries and transgenic nanobody-producing animals. The phage display method encompasses immunization, library preparation, cloning into phagemid vectors, and transformation into an appropriate E. coli strain. This process is followed by panning against the target antigen, and subsequent washing and elution. In the case of nanobody-producing transgenic animals, the methodology includes immunization, direct B cell screening, and cloning, succeeded by in vitro evaluation. Ultimately, antigen-specific nanobodies are harvested using diverse expression platforms, including plants, bacteria, yeast, and mammalian cells. This figure was crafted using BioRender.com.

Multivalent Constructs of Nanobodies

Nanobodies, owing to their unique properties, have demonstrated significant potential for applications in infectious diseases (Figure 2). Nevertheless, their low molecular weight often leads to a short half-life, hindering long-term treatment. This challenge can be partially addressed by constructing multivalent nanobodies (Nbs). This construction method is both simple and versatile, thanks to nanobodies' fully hydrophilic surfaces and lack of light chains. This enables the construction of bivalent or multivalent Nbs using linker peptides such as the flexible glycine-serine (G4S) linker. This linker can tandemly connect different Nbs to form bivalent or multivalent molecules, often enhancing their affinity or providing diverse specificity [35-37]. Additionally, multivalent Nbs can be constructed using chemical bonds formed by amino acid interactions, such as disulfide bonds. Multivalent constructs not only maintain their physicochemical properties, including high solubility, yield, and stability, but also demonstrate potent neutralizing activity against pseudoviruses even after lyophilization and aerosolization. This makes them suitable for various drug delivery approaches [38]. The affinity and viral blocking efficacy of multivalent Nbs can be significantly increased when constructed using homologous Nbs, making them promising for blocking viral mutations that evade detection by binding to multiple epitopes within the SARS-CoV-2 RBD [39]. Nanobodies Targeting SARS-CoV-2 The receptor-binding domain (RBD) of SARS-CoV-2 facilitates viral entry into cells by binding to the human angiotensin-converting enzyme 2 (ACE2) receptor. Consequently, the RBD is a crucial target for immunotherapy. Several researchers have constructed nanobodies that bind with high affinity to the RBD, blocking further invasion [39-42]. Applications in Other Infectious Diseases Multivalent Nbs have also shown promising applications in other infectious diseases. Bispecific Nbs targeting HIV have exhibited significant neutralizing effects [43]. Trimeric nanobody ALX-0171 has undergone clinical trials, targeting Respiratory syncytial virus (RSV) with potent effects [38, 44, 45]. There have also been innovative constructions of bispecific nanobodies against influenza A virus [46], Shigella spp. [47], Rift Valley Fever virus (RVFV), and Schmallenberg virus (SBV) [48]. Challenges and Future Directions Despite the advanced performance of polyvalent Nbs and the sophistication of antibody engineering techniques, the optimal design of nanobody combinations and forms remains a complex endeavor. The functionality of nanobodies can vary greatly depending on their construction, and determining the best therapeutic approach may require further investigation [48-51]. Although there are promising developments in the field, the creation of multivalent Nbs with optimal performance demands substantial ongoing research and experimentation. In conclusion, multivalent nanobodies represent an exciting frontier in the treatment of infectious diseases. Their versatility, efficacy, and adaptability offer a wide range of possibilities for therapeutic applications. Further exploration and innovation in this domain may yield even more potent and flexible tools for combating a myriad of health challenges.

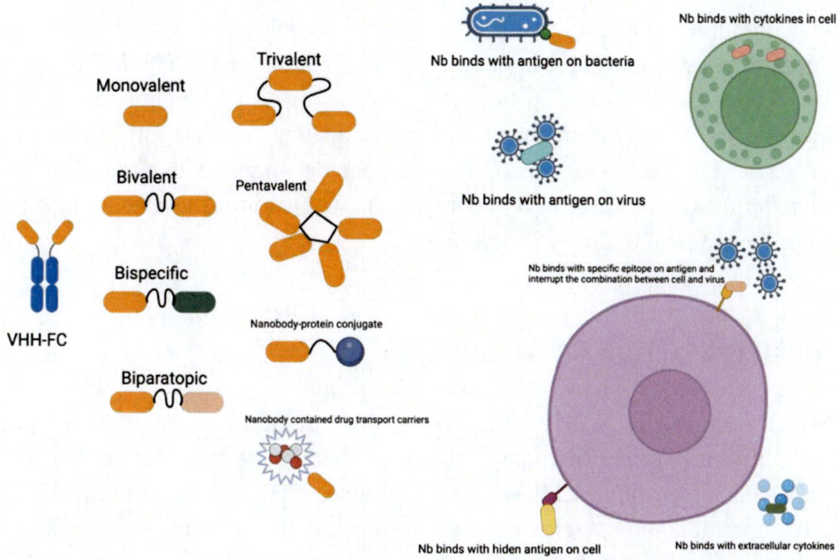

Figure 2. "Utilization of Nanobodies in Combating Human Infectious Diseases". This illustration depicts the application of nanobodies and their derivatives in targeting infectious diseases. This figure was crafted using BioRender.com.

Nanobody Conjugates and Combinations

Nanobodies are highly adaptable and lend themselves well to modification and engineering. In various applications, fusion proteins of nanobodies are crafted to amplify therapeutic impacts. One common form is the VHH-Fc, where a nanobody is linked to the IgG Fc region. This construction not only extends the half-life of the molecule but also enhances its antiviral effects and facilitates Fc-mediated effector functions [52-54]. Research by Nick S et al. revealed that nanobody fusion proteins containing Fc had a more potent effect against the influenza virus [54]. Furthermore, the VHH-Fc form targeting Mycoplasma hominis demonstrated effective preventive and therapeutic results in mouse models [52]. Nanobodies also hold potential in combination with drug molecules to create therapeutic synergy. For many drugs, ensuring specific transport to the intended therapeutic target remains a significant challenge. Take small RNA-based molecules, for instance; they often suffer from inefficient cellular uptake due to their negative charge. These molecules generally rely on their inherent hydrophilicity and small molecular weight for in vivo delivery, leading to low transport efficiency, increased drug consumption, and severe side effects [55]. Nanobodies, with their flexible structure and function, can serve as excellent tailored vehicles for these molecules. As illustrated in Figure 2, proteins fused with nanobodies can be specifically transported to their target locations, enhancing therapeutic efficacy. The following sections will provide concrete examples of how nanobodies can be harnessed in conjunction with various therapeutic agents to improve medical treatment outcomes.

Small Interfering RNAs (siRNAs)

Small interfering RNAs (siRNAs) are pivotal in regulating post-transcriptional gene silencing, and their therapeutic application has been validated for treating localized regions in vivo, such as within intraocular and intracerebral disorders. However, the systemic delivery of therapeutic siRNAs encounters substantial limitations. Therapeutic molecules, formulated by coupling siRNA molecules with cell-penetrating peptides, are often too small, causing rapid clearance by the kidneys and rendering the therapy ineffective. Chimeric constructs based on Nb (nanobodies), such as VHH-siRNA, specifically target siRNA inhibitors to deploy their inhibitory function and exhibit promising potential for treating various diseases. C-X-C chemokinc receptor type 4 (CXCR4) is abundantly expressed on CD4+ T lymphocytes, notably those infected with HIV. The interaction between CXCR4 and its natural ligand plays a crucial role in initiating internalization. A breakthrough study by Cunha-Santos et al. leveraged nanobodies targeting CXCR4 to construct chimeras that facilitate siRNA translocation across membranes. This innovative approach has been shown to silence HIV viral transcription effectively and inhibit viral infectivity [55], providing a clear example of how nanobodies can contribute to targeted therapeutic strategies.

Immunotoxins

Immunotoxins are protein-based therapeutics that, once bound to specific cell-surface antigens, can internalize into the target cell and exert therapeutic effects [56]. The strategic conjugation of nanobodies with immunotoxins has enabled targeted delivery, optimizing the killing efficiency of virally infected cells. One illustrative example involves glycoprotein D (gD2), a critical molecule found on the vaginal herpes simplex virus (HSV-2), which plays a vital role in viral infection. Researchers have fused the Nb R33, which specifically targets gD2 but lacks virus-neutralizing ability, with the cytotoxic domain of Pseudomonas aeruginosa exotoxin A. This fusion created an immunotoxin that was not only shown to augment toxin killing but also to eradicate virally infected cells more efficiently compared to the cytotoxic domain alone [57]. Additionally, apolipoprotein L-I (apoL-I) has demonstrated the ability to lyse African trypanosomes. A recombinant immunotoxin, constructed by coupling NbAn33 (targeting trypanosomes) to apoL-I, was successful in fully eradicating the parasite in mouse models. Remarkably, this therapeutic approach was achieved without causing any detrimental side effects [58]. This fusion technology, incorporating nanobodies with immunotoxins, represents an exciting advancement in targeted therapeutics, opening doors for more precise and potent interventions against various infectious diseases.

Drug Molecules

Some drug molecules face challenges in directly fusing with nanobodies to form fusion proteins for co-targeting therapeutic targets. In these cases, nanobodies can be constructed as carriers to transport these drugs. The targeted delivery facilitated by nanobodies can reduce the therapeutic dose, enhance efficacy, minimize side effects, and circumvent resistance mechanisms stemming from surface transporter protein mutations. A prime example of this technology's application is in the treatment of African trypanosomiasis, a lethal disease where continuous antigenic variation hinders the host immune response and the application of vaccine immunization. Concurrently, mutations in surface drug transport proteins can fast-track drug resistance. Juan D. Unciti-Broceta et al. created a drug nanocarrier composed of polymeric nanoparticles encapsulated with nanobodies, targeting the surface of trypanosomes, and containing the trypanocidal drug pentamidine. This innovative approach allows the drug to enter trypanosomes via endocytosis, bypassing classical cell surface transport proteins. In vitro experiments demonstrated superior efficacy of the pentamidine-loaded nanoparticles compared to pentamidine alone. Moreover, in vivo mouse models showed successful treatment with a significantly lower drug dose [59].

Vaccine Antigens

Nanobodies can be paired with vaccines to augment therapeutic efficacy. For example, anti-rabies nanobodies have been combined with post-exposure prophylaxis (PEP) vaccines for rabies. This approach extended the median survival time in intranasally infected mice and increased survival rates compared to nanobody treatment alone [60]. Targeted delivery of antigens to antigen-presenting cells (APCs) can further enhance immune effects. Examples include the creation of virus-like particles (VLPs) that induce humoral immunity against papillomavirus (HPV) and the development of a SARS-CoV-2 vaccine by fusing a nanobody with the SARS-CoV-2 spike RBD. These innovative solutions elicit potent immune responses and offer promising treatments for HPV+ patients and COVID-19 [61, 62]. Furthermore, Amcheslavsky et al. proposed utilizing nanobodies' recognition of conserved epitopes to reverse engineer vaccines aimed at Enterotoxigenic Escherichia coli (ETEC). By identifying nanobodies that recognize a conserved epitope in the ETEC adhesion proteins, they demonstrated that rational vaccine design based on this epitope could lead to more effective disease prevention [63]. In summary, the utilization of nanobodies in the transport of drug molecules and enhancement of vaccine antigens illustrates an exciting frontier in targeted therapeutics. These novel approaches hold significant potential for the treatment and prevention of a wide array of diseases, advancing the capabilities of modern medicine.

Nanobody Targeting Receptor Proteins

Receptor proteins within the human body represent promising targets for immunotherapy in treating infectious diseases. Traditional antibodies can bind receptor proteins, thereby preventing pathogenic invasion. However, targeting specific multifunctional receptors involved in viral infection and essential physiological processes poses a challenge. Conventional antibodies often recognize chemical groups, peptides, and epitopes located on large protein surfaces, making it difficult for them to target small, concealed epitopes without disrupting other physiological responses. As a result, direct targeting using conventional antibodies can lead to serious side effects [64, 65]. Nanobodies offer a more nuanced approach. They can effectively bind to receptors and act with precision. For example, Thomas J et al. identified nanobodies that bind to human ACE2, blocking the interaction of the receptor-binding domain (RBD) and ACE2 with high affinity [66]. Furthermore, the longer CDR3 region of nanobodies, forming finger-like extensions, allows them to bind small hidden epitopes, a feature not accessible to traditional antibodies [65, 67]. This capability enables nanobodies to selectively bind multifunctional epitopes on receptors, blocking disease-related pathways without disturbing the receptor's typical function, thus minimizing treatment side effects. CXCR4, a G protein-coupled receptor (GPCR), exemplifies the targeted approach enabled by nanobodies. Involved in numerous physiological responses, CXCR4 is also a key co-receptor for HIV entry into CD4-positive T cells, making it a valuable target for HIV therapy. Traditional drugs targeting CXCR4 may interfere with its normal functions, leading to undesired consequences. In contrast, nanobodies can provide precise targeting, effectively inhibiting HIV while preserving the receptor's regular physiological roles [68]. A study by Van Hout et al. identified a nanobody recognizing an epitope on CXCR4 distinct from other ligand-binding sites, demonstrating the potential for nanobodies to minimize immunotherapy side effects [64]. In conclusion, the ability of nanobodies to target concealed and multifunctional epitopes on receptor proteins offers a refined therapeutic strategy, maintaining the balance between effective treatment and preservation of normal physiological functions. This approach expands the possibilities of immunotherapy, with the potential to enhance both the efficacy and safety of treatments for a variety of infectious diseases.

Nanobody Targeting of Pathogens

During the life cycle of pathogens within the host organism, numerous stages, such as cell attachment and entry, replication and regulation, transcription and translation, and virion assembly, provide a multitude of potential targets for intervention [69, 70]. Pathogens often exhibit diverse epitopes with low homology to human proteins, making them appealing targets for immunotherapy. However, treating infectious diseases using immunotherapy has its challenges. One significant obstacle is the intricate spatial conformations that many key epitopes on pathogens assume. These conformations are frequently hidden under other molecules, like glycoproteins, making them evasive to recognition by conventional antibodies [71, 72]. Such hidden epitopes include those that facilitate pathogen entry into human cells or those that are crucial virulence factors. These complexities hinder the development of effective therapeutic antibodies following pathogen infection. Additionally, the continuous emergence of new variations presents an enormous challenge to infection therapy, particularly in combating viral infections. Most antibodies targeting epitopes on pathogens are unable to offer sufficient protection against different subtypes or future strains. Nevertheless, antibodies capable of broad neutralization across various viral subtypes have been identified. These antibodies bind to highly conserved viral epitopes, though such antibodies are rare since viruses often conceal these essential pathogenic determinants, making them challenging to detect with conventional antibodies. Nanobodies offer an innovative solution to these challenges. With their lower molecular weight and extended CDR3 region, nanobodies can achieve higher affinity and recognition ability, rendering them more adept at binding to these concealed and conserved epitopes [73-75]. Unlike traditional antibodies, nanobodies can access pockets or clefts where conserved epitopes are hidden. Therefore, nanobodies are anticipated to be a superior strategy for targeting pathogens across various subtypes or even future emergent strains. In conclusion, nanobodies open up new avenues in the field of infectious disease treatment. Their unique structure and ability to recognize otherwise inaccessible epitopes present a promising option for the development of therapies that can adapt to the evolving landscape of pathogenic threats.

Norovirus

Nanobodies exhibit a multifaceted approach in inhibiting pathogen infection by mechanisms such as obstructing viral entry into cells or neutralizing toxins secreted by pathogens, thereby preventing harm to the body. A pertinent example is human norovirus, a significant causative agent of gastroenteritis for which vaccines or antivirals have not yet been developed. Structural analyses of norovirus have identified that the protruding (P) domains contain the main determinants for host binding factors, with histo-blood group antigens (HBGAs) playing a crucial role as binding factors within the P domain. A comprehensive screening of a large nanobody library against norovirus yielded an assortment of nanobodies that target different epitopes. Interestingly, some of these nanobodies directly coincide with HBGA binding sites and can compete with the receptors,

Table 1. Representative nanobodies for infectious diseases

Nanobody	Disease	Target	Structure features	References
VHH-72	SARS-CoV-2	RBD	Bivalent, VHH-Fc	[76, 77]
Nb15-NbH-Nb15	SARS-CoV-2	RBD	tri- valent with albumin specific Nb	[78]
Nanosota-1C-Fc	SARS-CoV-2	RBD	Monovalent VHH-Fc	[79]
Nb21	SARS-CoV-2	RBD	Monovalent	[80, 81]
Sb#15, Sb#68	SARS-CoV-2	RBD	Monovalent, bivalent	[82]
1B-3F-Fc, 3F- 1B-2A-Fc, 1B-3F-2A-Fc	SARS-CoV-2	RBD	Bispecific, trispecific VHH-Fc	[83]
n3113	SARS-CoV-2	RBD	Monovalent	[84]
RBD1i13, RBD3i17, RBD6id, RBD10i10, RBD10i14, RBD11i12	SARS-CoV-2	RBD	Monovalent, bivalent VHH-Fc	[85]
WNb 2, WNb 7, WNb 15, WNb 36	SARS-CoV-2	RBD	Monovalent, bivalent; VHH-Fc	[86]
MR3	SARS-CoV-2	RBD	Bivalent Nb; bispecific Nb; VHH-Fc	[87]
D7 , D3	Ehrlichia infection	T4SS effector	CPP-Nb conjugation	[88]
CeVICA	SARS-CoV-2	RBD	Nb-His tag	[30]
Fu2	SARS-CoV-2	RBD	Bispecific; bivalent; trivalent; VHH-Fc	[89]
125s	chronic hepatitis B infection	hepatitis B surface antigen	VHH-Fc	[90]
/	Fungal Keratitis	Dectin 1	Nb-His tag	[91]
VUN100	Latent human cytomegalovirus (HCMV) infection	signaling of the viral receptor US28	Nb–photosensitizer conjugates; bivalent Nb; Nb-His tag;	[92, 93]
Nb113 and IB10	Shiga toxin-producing Escherichia coli (STEC)	the B subunit of Shiga toxin 2 (Stx2B) and the C terminus of Intimin (IntC280)	Bispecific Nb	[94, 95]
Nb13	Mal de Río Cuarto virus (MRCV)	the major viral viroplasm component, P9-1.	Nb-alkaline phosphatase; Nb-eGFP fusion	[96]

Table 1. (Continued)

Nanobody	Disease	Target	Structure features	References
NB7-14	Influenza H7N9 virus	HA	Bivalent Nb	[97]
C5, H3, C1, F2	SARS-CoV-2	RBD	Homotrimers Nb; VHH-Fc	[98]
aEv6	Ebola Virus	EBOV GP	Nb-Fc	[99]
aRBD-2, aRBD-3, aRBD-5, aRBD-7, aRBD-41, aRBD-42, and aRBD-54.	SARS-CoV-2	RBD	Bispecific Nb; Nb-His tag; Nb-Fc;	[41]
Nb1	bovine viral diarrhea virus	The nonstructural protein 5	Nb-eGFP fusion	[100]
NbCXCR4	human immunodeficiency virus	CXCR4	fuse Nb to an anti-fluorescein (FITC) scFv responsible for carrying the FITC-labeled siRNA	[101, 102].
NbMS10	Middle East respiratory syndrome (MERS) coronavirus (MERS-CoV)	RBD	bivalent Nb trimer Nb Nb-His tag Nb-Fc	[103, 104]
SNB02	Severe fever with thrombocytopenia syndrome virus* (SFTSV)	the extracellular domain of SFTSV Gn (sGn)	Nb-Fc	[105]

thereby blocking virion binding sites. This competitive binding mechanism is not the only way that nanobodies work to neutralize the virus. In addition to their receptor-blocking capability, some nanobodies inflict structural damage on the virions, further inhibiting their ability to bind to host cells. By binding at a dimeric interface on the lower side of the P dimer, these nanobodies disrupt structural changes in the capsid that are associated with binding cofactors. What's more, the nanobodies can induce conformational rearrangements in various P domain loops, leading to particle aggregation and interference within the HBGA binding pocket [69, 106]. This innovative approach to norovirus inhibition was also demonstrated by Kerstin Ruoff and colleagues, who showed that nanobodies could target different sites and inhibit infection through multiple mechanisms. The therapeutic effects were further enhanced by a combination of treatments utilizing different nanobodies that recognize multiple epitopes [107]. This intricate network of mechanisms not only highlights the versatility of nanobodies in therapeutic interventions but also paves the way for exploring their potential applications against other infectious diseases.

Plasmodium Falciparum

Plasmodium falciparum, the causative agent of placental malaria, leads to severe consequences for both mothers and children. The infection process is mediated by the plasmodium-expressed protein Variant surface antigen 2-CSA (VAR2CSA), which adheres to chondroitin sulfate A (CSA) in the human placenta, resulting in the accumulation of infected erythrocytes (IE). Consequently, this interaction becomes a critical target for therapeutic intervention. While antibodies aimed at the CSA-binding epitopes on VAR2CSA can effectively block this interaction and thereby prevent the adhesion of IE, the task is complicated by the size and structural complexity of VAR2CSA. Specifically, the epitope region responsible for CSA binding is small and cryptic, rendering the identification of targeted antibodies particularly challenging. In this context, nanobodies offer a compelling solution. Unlike conventional antibodies, nanobodies are capable of recognizing cryptic and conformational epitopes that remain inaccessible to traditional antibody approaches. Furthermore, they interact with smaller immunogenic epitopes, making them an effective alternative for targeting nonimmune dominant regions. In a pioneering study by Sisse B. Ditlev et al., alpacas were directly immunized with the full-length VAR2CSA (FV2), bypassing the immunodominant domains of VAR2CSA, to screen for Nbs specifically targeting this protein. This innovative approach led to the identification of nanobodies that recognized a range of nonimmune dominant and concealed epitopes on VAR2CSA, including those in the CSA-binding region [108]. These findings are not only an essential advancement in our understanding of the molecular mechanisms underlying placental malaria but also represent a promising step towards the development of more targeted and effective diagnostics and treatments. The discovery of these specific nanobodies highlights the potential for employing similar strategies in the battle against other complex diseases, reflecting the versatility and promise of nanobody-based therapies.

Listeria Monocytogenes

Listeria monocytogenes is a food-borne pathogen that poses a high risk to pregnant women and may lead to termination of fetal development. The interaction of internalin B (InlB) with the c-Met receptor is essential for bacteria to cross the placental barrier in pregnant women. InlB is hidden in the peptidoglycan layer, which is difficult for conventional antibodies to bind and inhibit. A previous study showed that Nbs are small enough to penetrate the listeria cell to bind the target protein. They can bind to the c-Met receptor-binding site on InlB with high affinity and competitively inhibit bacterial invasion, preventing fetal infection [72].

Seasonal influenza viruses persist in causing global epidemics annually, leading to substantial morbidity, mortality, and societal distress. Compounding the challenge, the rapid accumulation of genetic mutations means that influenzas frequently evolve, presenting an array of subtypes. These ongoing mutations make novel influenza pandemics both recurrent and unpredictable, sparking serious concern about potential future pandemics. Consequently, the development of effective prophylactic and therapeutic interventions is an urgent necessity. Broadly neutralizing antibodies against influenza represent an appealing strategy for developing a wide-ranging treatment against diverse influenza viruses. The M2 ion channel, which has an extracellular domain conserved across all human influenza A viruses, provides an intriguing potential target for broad-spectrum therapy. However, the sparse presence and low immunogenicity of M2 molecules on influenza viral particles have hindered the development of vaccines targeting this epitope. In an innovative approach, the nanobody M2-7A has been shown to target the

M2 ion channel on the virus with robust affinity. This nanobody exhibits potent neutralizing activity against numerous subtypes of influenza A viruses, signifying remarkable broad-spectrum neutralization potential [73]. Additionally, Hemagglutinin (HA), an essential factor in mediating virus-host cell receptor binding and membrane fusion, has emerged as a key target for anti-influenza drugs and vaccines [75]. Notably, Hufton et al. have identified several nanobodies that target the HA protein domain of influenza viruses, revealing substantial cross-neutralization potential. One particularly promising nanobody, R1A-B6, has demonstrated exceptional cross-neutralizing capability, binding to H1N1 and H5N1 with IC50 values in the single-digit nanomolar range. Further research indicates that engineering these nanobodies into bivalent or multivalent forms may further enhance their neutralizing activity and therapeutic efficacy [109, 110]. In summary, the discovery and development of nanobodies targeting key viral structures present a compelling pathway to broad-spectrum influenza treatment. These advancements underscore the importance of continued exploration and innovation in this field, offering hope for more effective and versatile interventions against influenza viruses and potential preparedness against future pandemics.

HIV

The relentless challenge of human immunodeficiency virus type 1 (HIV-1) demands innovative approaches to both treatment and prevention. A key to unlocking new therapies lies within the GP41 glycoprotein of the virus, specifically a highly conserved segment found within the membrane-proximal external region (MPER). This region is recognized as a common target for HIV neutralizing antibodies. However, the MPER's unique spatial conformation, coupled with the virus's sophisticated evasion strategies, has rendered conventional immunization protocols using gp41 peptides or protein immunization largely ineffective in producing broad-spectrum cross-neutralizing antibodies that target MPER. In a notable advancement, some researchers have immunized alpacas with gp41-MPER proteoliposomes, leading to the identification of the MPER-specific nanobody 2H10. This particular nanobody is adept at binding to epitopes with low nanomolar affinity across various particle conformations. Through detailed crystal structure studies, it has been revealed that 2H10 possesses an extended CDR3 region with a solvent-exposed tryptophan at its tip. The innovative construction of a bivalent nanobody, termed bi-2H10, has yielded even more promising results. By simultaneously binding two GP41 trimers or interacting with two GP41 molecules on the same trimer, bi-2H10 has achieved enhanced immunosuppression [71]. The discoveries related to 2H10 open an intriguing path towards more effective treatment strategies for HIV-1. By exploring the potential of nanobodies targeting the conserved segments of the virus, researchers are inching closer to solutions that could contribute substantially to the ongoing battle against HIV. These advances also underscore the broader potential of nanobodies in tackling other complex and evasive pathogens.

HPV

The dynamic and often stealthy behavior of many pathogens—invading cells, proliferating within them, and triggering a cascade of intracellular reactions—often leads to extensive bodily harm while skillfully evading external immune mechanisms. This presents a complex challenge for conventional antibody therapies, which often struggle to penetrate cellular barriers and maintain functionality within cells. In contrast, the unique attributes of nanobodies have unveiled promising new pathways for immunological intervention. Due to their small molecular size, nanobodies can be engineered as "intracellular antibodies," or intrabodies, targeting intracellular antigens. This enables them to inhibit these antigens' functions with precision, thereby exerting potent immune effects. Among the exciting initial successes in this realm is the application of nanobody-based intrabodies in the treatment of human papillomavirus (HPV), a persistent infection that can lead to the development of cervical cancer. The E6 and E7 proteins of HPV16, a prevalent strain of HPV in humans, are notably implicated in tumor aggressiveness. Researchers have identified specific nanobodies, namely Nb9 and Nb2, that selectively bind to E6 and E7. When expressed in HPV16-positive cells as intracellular Nbs, both Nb9 and Nb2 were found to inhibit tumor cell proliferation in vitro. Encouraged by these results, further in vivo studies using animal models were conducted to explore the therapeutic potential of Nb9 alone, and in combination with Nb2. Both modalities demonstrated significant inhibition of tumor growth, with the combination therapy proving more effective. These experimental outcomes have illuminated the promising value of nanobodies as intrabodies in treating HPV-associated lesions, reinforcing the broader potential of this approach in targeting intracellular pathogens. The lessons learned from these endeavors stand as compelling evidence that nanobodies may offer a powerful new weapon in the ongoing battle against challenging intracellular infections [111, 112].

Other Pathogens

Treating infections caused by intracellular obligate pathogens poses significant challenges due to the complexities of targeting intracellular mechanisms and developing effective delivery systems. However, innovative approaches using nanobodies are making inroads into these difficult areas.

Ehrlichia chaffeensis: This intracellular bacterium uses Ehrlichia translocated factor-1 (Etf-1) as its primary virulence factor. Secreted Etf-1 latches onto mitochondria in host cells, preventing apoptosis (programmed cell death) and enabling the bacterium's survival and replication within the host. Remarkably, nanobodies have been discovered to enter cells and specifically interfere with Etf-1's mitochondrial localization. This action disrupts the function of Etf-1 and successfully prevents Chaffeensis infection in both cellular and mouse models [88].

Porcine Reproductive and Respiratory Syndrome Virus (PRRSV): PRRSV is an antigenically diverse virus that makes traditional antibody targeting challenging. However, nanobodies aimed at specific epitopes of PRRSV have proven effective in blocking or entirely preventing PRRSV replication. They achieve this by inhibiting the viral genome's replication and transcription, and by stopping virus-induced cell damage [74].

Campylobacter jejuni and E. coli.: Nanobodies that target conserved epitopes on these bacteria's major outer membrane proteins also demonstrate promising therapeutic and diagnostic applications [113].

Nanobody Binding Regulators

Nanobodies play a critical role in binding to immune factors within the body, actively participating in the immune regulation of diseases. Their involvement is particularly noteworthy in the following contexts:

1. *Septic Shock*: Septic shock is a leading cause of mortality among intensive care patients, making the prevention and treatment of this condition a priority in medical care. A key factor in this disease is

Macrophage Migration Inhibitory Factor (MIF), an upstream immunomodulatory mediator released by myeloid cells, pivotal in the mechanisms leading to infections and septic shock. Targeting MIF offers an attractive therapeutic approach. In this context, nanobodies have emerged as powerful tools. They can bind to MIF with nanomolar affinities, significantly inhibiting MIF activity. This not only reduces the MIF-induced effects but also curtails endotoxic shock-mediated lethality in mouse models, offering promising therapeutic prospects [114].

2. *HIV Regulation*: The Regulator of Expression of Virion Protein (REV) serves as an essential transcriptional activator in HIV gene replication. REV mediates the transport of HIV mRNAs from the nucleus to the cytoplasm by multimerizing on the secondary stem–loop structure of viral intron-containing mRNAs. A specially-designed nanobody, Nb190, has been shown to robustly inhibit REV multimerization, thereby hindering the production and spread of new HIV viruses. The work of Boons et al. illustrates the potential of this approach. By directly transfecting plasmids containing the Nb190 sequence into cells and constructing cell lines stably expressing Nb190, they demonstrated that these cells were relatively protected against virus-induced cytopathological changes. Moreover, sequence analysis revealed that the sites targeted by Nb190 in REV were conserved across major HIV-1 subtypes, indicating that Nb190 might offer a broad-spectrum inhibitory effect against different HIV-1 subtypes [115].

These developments in nanobody binding regulators present innovative paths for both understanding and treating complex immunological diseases. The applications in septic shock and HIV regulation emphasize the potential of nanobodies as specialized agents capable of precise targeting and modulation, ushering in exciting possibilities for future medical interventions.

Conclusion

Infectious diseases pose a profound threat to global human health. The unchecked proliferation of COVID-19, along with other infectious maladies, has given rise to more stringent demands for the prevention and treatment of such diseases. Our examination of recent studies reveals that nanobodies—

along with multi-specific drugs and imaging reagents constructed with nanobodies—present a promising alternative therapeutic avenue to combat both bacterial and viral outbreaks. Nanobodies are characterized by their superb tissue penetration, high affinity, adaptable structure, and cost-efficient expression system. These attributes offer innovative concepts and breakthroughs for the prevention and treatment of infectious diseases. The potential applications of nanobodies are extensive and encompass various aspects of infectious diseases, including the inhibition of viral transcriptional replication and cellular entry, the neutralization of viral toxins, the stimulation of the human immune system, and the destruction of virus-infected cells. The attention directed towards nanobodies is escalating, particularly concerning their roles in preventing and treating bacterial toxins, traditional malignant infectious diseases, and acute infectious maladies. Recent amassed clinical and experimental data propose that multimeric and functionalized molecules constructed with nanobodies may become an essential component of future diagnostic and therapeutic reagents, particularly in the context of infectious diseases. However, as a novel form of antibody, there remain many complexities to unravel before we can translate the foundational research on nanobodies into applied products and subsequently move towards clinical implementation. The realization of this goal necessitates the collaborative efforts of future researchers. In conclusion, the employment of nanobodies for the prevention, detection, and treatment of a wide array of infectious diseases stands to enhance human life and health. This approach not only offers a tailored response to public health crises triggered by infectious diseases but also promotes a more economical and efficient public health system.

References

[1] Tokuhara, D., et al., Rice-based oral antibody fragment prophylaxis and therapy against rotavirus infection. *J Clin Invest,* 2013. **123**(9): p. 3829-38.

[2] Sarker, S.A., et al., Anti-Rotavirus Protein Reduces Stool Output in Infants With Diarrhea: A Randomized Placebo-Controlled Trial. *Gastroenterology,* 2013. **145**(4): p. 740-748.e8.

[3] Hamerscasterman, C., et al., Naturally-Occurring Antibodies Devoid of Light-Chains. *Nature,* 1993. **363**(6428): p. 446-448.

[4] Salvador, J.P., L. Vilaplana, and M.P. Marco, Nanobody: outstanding features for diagnostic and therapeutic applications. *Analytical and Bioanalytical Chemistry,* 2019. **411**(9): p. 1703-1713.

[5] De Genst, E., et al., Molecular basis for the preferential cleft recognition by dromedary heavy-chain antibodies. *Proceedings of the National Academy of Sciences of the United States of America,* 2006. **103**(12): p. 4586-4591.
[6] Steeland, S., R.E. Vandenbroucke, and C. Libert, Nanobodies as therapeutics: big opportunities for small antibodies. *Drug Discovery Today,* 2016. **21**(7): p. 1076-1113.
[7] Zavrtanik, U., et al., Structural Basis of Epitope Recognition by Heavy-Chain Camelid Antibodies. *Journal of Molecular Biology,* 2018. **430**(21): p. 4369-4386.
[8] Dumoulin, M., et al., Single-domain antibody fragments with high conformational stability. *Protein Science,* 2002. **11**(3): p. 500-515.
[9] Li, M., et al., Selection by phage display of nanobodies directed against hypoxia inducible factor-1 alpha (HIF-1 alpha). *Biotechnology and Applied Biochemistry,* 2015. **62**(6): p. 738-745.
[10] Omidfar, K. and M. Daneshpour, Advances in phage display technology for drug discovery. *Expert Opinion on Drug Discovery,* 2015. **10**(6): p. 651-669.
[11] Almagro, J.C. and J. Fransson, Humanization of antibodies. *Front Biosci,* 2008. **13**: p. 1619-33.
[12] De Genst, E., et al., Chemical basis for the affinity maturation of a camel single domain antibody. *J Biol Chem,* 2004. **279**(51): p. 53593-601.
[13] Vincke, C., et al., General Strategy to Humanize a Camelid Single-domain Antibody and Identification of a Universal Humanized Nanobody Scaffold. *Journal of Biological Chemistry,* 2009. **284**(5): p. 3273-3284.
[14] Liu, W.S., et al., Recent advances in the selection and identification of antigen-specific nanobodies. *Molecular Immunology,* 2018. **96**: p. 37-47.
[15] Janssens, R., et al., Generation of heavy-chain-only antibodies in mice. *Proc Natl Acad Sci U S A,* 2006. **103**(41): p. 15130-5.
[16] Liu, B. and D. Yang, Easily Established and Multifunctional Synthetic Nanobody Libraries as Research Tools. Int J Mol Sci, 2022. **23**(3).
[17] Muyldermans, S., A guide to: generation and design of nanobodies. *Febs j,* 2021. **288**(7): p. 2084-2102.
[18] Yan, J.R., et al., Characterization and applications of Nanobodies against human procalcitonin selected from a novel naive Nanobody phage display library. *Journal of Nanobiotechnology,* 2015. **13**.
[19] Muyldermans, S., Nanobodies: Natural Single-Domain Antibodies. *Annual Review of Biochemistry,* Vol 82, 2013. **82**: p. 775-797.
[20] Koide, A., et al., Exploring the capacity of minimalist protein interfaces: interface energetics and affinity maturation to picomolar KD of a single-domain antibody with a flat paratope. *Journal of molecular biology,* 2007. **373**(4): p. 941-953.
[21] Lecocq, Q., et al., Theranostics in immuno-oncology using nanobody derivatives. *Theranostics,* 2019. **9**(25): p. 7772-7791.
[22] Makvandi-Nejad, S., et al., Selection and expression of recombinant single domain antibodies from a hyper-immunized library against the hapten azoxystrobin. *Journal of Immunological Methods,* 2011. **373**(1-2): p. 8-18.
[23] Ezzine, A., et al., Efficient expression of the anti-AahI' scorpion toxin nanobody under a new functional form in a Pichia pastoris system. 2012. **59**(1): p. 15-21.

[24] Gorlani, A., H. de Haard, and T. Verrips, Expression of VHHs in Saccharomyces cerevisiae, in *Single Domain Antibodies: Methods and Protocols,* D. Saerens and S. Muyldermans, Editors. 2012, Humana Press: Totowa, NJ. p. 277-286.

[25] de Marco, A., Recombinant expression of nanobodies and nanobody-derived immunoreagents. Protein Expr Purif, 2020. **172**: p. 105645.

[26] Djender, S., et al., Bacterial cytoplasm as an effective cell compartment for producing functional VHH-based affinity reagents and Camelidae IgG-like recombinant antibodies. *Microb Cell Fact,* 2014. **13**: p. 140.

[27] Liu, Z.-h., et al., Comparison of three commonly used fusion tags for the expression of nanobodies in the cytoplasm of Escherichia coli. *Biotechnology & Biotechnological Equipment*, 2018. **32**(2): p. 462-469.

[28] Hoogenboom, H.R., Selecting and screening recombinant antibody libraries. *Nature Biotechnology,* 2005. **23**(9): p. 1105-1116.

[29] McMahon, C., et al., Yeast surface display platform for rapid discovery of conformationally selective nanobodies. *Nat Struct Mol Biol,* 2018. **25**(3): p. 289-296.

[30] Chen, X., et al., A cell-free nanobody engineering platform rapidly generates SARS-CoV-2 neutralizing nanobodies. *Nat Commun,* 2021. **12**(1): p. 5506.

[31] Virdi, V., et al., Orally fed seeds producing designer IgAs protect weaned piglets against enterotoxigenic Escherichia coli infection. *Proceedings of the National Academy of Sciences of the United States of America,* 2013. **110**(29): p. 11809-11814.

[32] Virdi, V., et al., Yeast-secreted, dried and food-admixed monomeric IgA prevents gastrointestinal infection in a piglet model. *Nature Biotechnology,* 2019. **37**(5): p. 527-+.

[33] Vanmarsenille, C., et al., In planta expression of nanobody-based designer chicken antibodies targeting Campylobacter. *Plos One,* 2018. **13**(9).

[34] Kalusche, S., et al., Lactobacilli Expressing Broadly Neutralizing Nanobodies against HIV-1 as Potential Vectors for HIV-1 Prophylaxis? *Vaccines,* 2020. **8**(4).

[35] Kostelny, S.A., M.S. Cole, and J.Y. Tso, Formation of a bispecific antibody by the use of leucine zippers. *J Immunol,* 1992. **148**(5): p. 1547-53.

[36] Els Conrath, K., et al., Camel single-domain antibodies as modular building units in bispecific and bivalent antibody constructs. *J Biol Chem,* 2001. **276**(10): p. 7346-50.

[37] Bannas, P., J. Hambach, and F. Koch-Nolte, Nanobodies and Nanobody-Based Human Heavy Chain Antibodies As Antitumor Therapeutics. *Frontiers in immunology,* 2017. **8**: p. 1603-1603.

[38] Detalle, L., et al., Generation and Characterization of ALX-0171, a Potent Novel Therapeutic Nanobody for the Treatment of Respiratory Syncytial Virus Infection. *Antimicrob Agents Chemother,* 2016. **60**(1): p. 6-13.

[39] Xiang, Y.F., et al., Versatile and multivalent nanobodies efficiently neutralize SARS-CoV-2. *Science,* 2020. **370**(6523): p. 1479-1484.

[40] Huo, J.D., et al., Neutralizing nanobodies bind SARS-CoV-2 spike RBD and block interaction with ACE2 (vol 27, pg 846, 2020). *Nature Structural & Molecular Biology,* 2021. **28**(3): p. 326-326.

[41] Ma, H., et al., Potent Neutralization of SARS-CoV-2 by Hetero-bivalent Alpaca Nanobodies Targeting the Spike Receptor-Binding Domain. *J Virol,* 2021. **95**(10).

[42] Dong, J.B., et al., Development of humanized tri-specific nanobodies with potent neutralization for SARS-CoV-2 (vol 10, 17806, 2020). *Scientific Reports,* 2021. **11**(1).

[43] Strokappe, N.M., et al., Super Potent Bispecific Llama VHH Antibodies Neutralize HIV via a Combination of gp41 and gp120 Epitopes. *Antibodies (Basel, Switzerland),* 2019. **8**(2): p. 38.

[44] Bruyn, S., et al., ALX-0171: Safety and therapeutic potential of an inhaled anti-RSV Nanobody. *RDD Europe* 2015, 2015. **1**: p. 37-48.

[45] Cunningham, S., et al., Nebulised ALX-0171 for respiratory syncytial virus lower respiratory tract infection in hospitalised children: a double-blind, randomised, placebo-controlled, phase 2b trial. *The Lancet Respiratory Medicine,* 2021. **9**(1): p. 21-32.

[46] De Vlieger, D., et al., Selective Engagement of FcγRIV by a M2e-Specific Single Domain Antibody Construct Protects Against Influenza A Virus Infection. *Frontiers in immunology,* 2019. **10**: p. 2920-2920.

[47] Barta, M.L., et al., Single-domain antibodies pinpoint potential targets within Shigella invasion plasmid antigen D of the needle tip complex for inhibition of type III secretion. *Journal of Biological Chemistry,* 2017. **292**(40): p. 16677-16687.

[48] Schreur, P.J.W., et al., Multimeric single-domain antibody complexes protect against bunyavirus infections. *Elife,* 2020. **9**.

[49] Iezzi, M.E., et al., Single-Domain Antibodies and the Promise of Modular Targeting in Cancer Imaging and Treatment. *Frontiers in Immunology,* 2018. **9**.

[50] De Tavernier, E., et al., High Throughput Combinatorial Formatting of PcrV Nanobodies for Efficient Potency Improvement. *Journal of Biological Chemistry,* 2016. **291**(29): p. 15243-15255.

[51] Koenig, P.A., et al., Structure-guided multivalent nanobodies block SARS-CoV-2 infection and suppress mutational escape. *Science,* 2021. **371**(6530): p. 691-+.

[52] Burmistrova, D.A., et al., Genetic Passive Immunization with Adenoviral Vector Expressing Chimeric Nanobody-Fc Molecules as Therapy for Genital Infection Caused by Mycoplasma hominis. *PLoS One,* 2016. **11**(3): p. e0150958.

[53] De Vlieger, D., et al., Single-Domain Antibodies and Their Formatting to Combat Viral Infections. *Antibodies (Basel, Switzerland),* 2018. **8**(1): p. 1.

[54] Laursen, N.S., et al., Universal protection against influenza infection by a multidomain antibody to influenza hemagglutinin. *Science,* 2018. **362**(6414): p. 598-602.

[55] Cunha-Santos, C., et al., Inhibition of HIV replication through siRNA carried by CXCR4-targeted chimeric nanobody. *Cellular and Molecular Life Sciences,* 2020. **77**(14): p. 2859-2870.

[56] Khirehgesh, M.R., et al., Immunotoxins and nanobody-based immunotoxins: review and update. *Journal of Drug Targeting,* 2021. **29**(8): p. 848-862.

[57] Geoghegan, E.M., et al., Antiviral Activity of a Single-Domain Antibody Immunotoxin Binding to Glycoprotein D of Herpes Simplex Virus 2. *Antimicrobial Agents and Chemotherapy,* 2015. **59**(1): p. 527-535.

[58] Baral, T.N., et al., Experimental therapy of African trypanosomiasis with a nanobody-conjugated human trypanolytic factor. *Nat Med,* 2006. **12**(5): p. 580-4.

[59] Unciti-Broceta, J.D., et al., Specific Cell Targeting Therapy Bypasses Drug Resistance Mechanisms in African Trypanosomiasis. *Plos Pathogens,* 2015. **11**(6).

[60] Terryn, S., et al., Post-exposure Treatment with Anti-rabies VHH and Vaccine Significantly Improves Protection of Mice from Lethal Rabies Infection. *Plos Neglected Tropical Diseases,* 2016. **10**(8).

[61] Woodham, A.W., et al., Nanobody-Antigen Conjugates Elicit HPV-Specific Antitumor Immune Responses. *Cancer immunology research,* 2018. **6**(7): p. 870-880.

[62] Pishesha, N., et al., A class II MHC-targeted vaccine elicits immunity against SARS-CoV-2 and its variants. *Proc Natl Acad Sci U S A,* 2021. **118**(44).

[63] Amcheslavsky, A., et al., Anti-CfaE nanobodies provide broad cross-protection against major pathogenic enterotoxigenic Escherichia coli strains, with implications for vaccine design. *Scientific Reports,* 2021. **11**(1): p. 2751.

[64] Van Hout, A., et al., CXCR4-targeting nanobodies differentially inhibit CXCR4 function and HIV entry. *Biochemical Pharmacology,* 2018. **158**: p. 402-412.

[65] Jovčevska, I. and S. Muyldermans, The Therapeutic Potential of Nanobodies. *BioDrugs: clinical immunotherapeutics, biopharmaceuticals and gene therapy,* 2020. **34**(1): p. 11-26.

[66] Esparza, T.J., et al., High affinity nanobodies block SARS-CoV-2 spike receptor binding domain interaction with human angiotensin converting enzyme. *Scientific Reports,* 2020. **10**(1): p. 22370.

[67] Schmitz, K.R., et al., Structural evaluation of EGFR inhibition mechanisms for nanobodies/VHH domains. *Structure,* 2013. **21**(7): p. 1214-24.

[68] Tian, S., et al., Distinct functional sites for human immunodeficiency virus type 1 and stromal cell-derived factor 1alpha on CXCR4 transmembrane helical domains. *Journal of virology,* 2005. **79**(20): p. 12667-12673.

[69] Koromyslova, A.D., et al., Nanobody-Mediated Neutralization Reveals an Achilles Heel for Norovirus. *Journal of Virology,* 2020. **94**(13).

[70] Tsukuda, S. and K. Watashi, Hepatitis B virus biology and life cycle. *Antiviral Research,* 2020. **182**.

[71] Lutje Hulsik, D., et al., A gp41 MPER-specific llama VHH requires a hydrophobic CDR3 for neutralization but not for antigen recognition. *PLoS pathogens,* 2013. **9**(3): p. e1003202-e1003202.

[72] King, M.T., et al., Structural basis of VHH-mediated neutralization of the food-borne pathogen Listeria monocytogenes. *Journal of Biological Chemistry,* 2018. **293**(35): p. 13626-13635.

[73] Wei, G.W., et al., Potent Neutralization of Influenza A Virus by a Single-Domain Antibody Blocking M2 Ion Channel Protein. *Plos One,* 2011. **6**(12).

[74] Liu, H.L., et al., An intracellularly expressed Nsp9-specific nanobody in MARC-145 cells inhibits porcine reproductive and respiratory syndrome virus replication. *Veterinary Microbiology,* 2015. **181**(3-4): p. 252-260.

[75] Gao, J.J., M. Gui, and Y. Xiang, Structural intermediates in the low pH-induced transition of influenza hemagglutinin. *Plos Pathogens,* 2020. **16**(11).

[76] Wrapp, D., et al., Structural Basis for Potent Neutralization of Betacoronaviruses by Single-Domain Camelid Antibodies. *Cell,* 2020. **181**(5): p. 1004-1015 e15.

[77] Scott, T.A., et al., Engineered extracellular vesicles directed to the spike protein inhibit SARS-CoV-2. *Mol Ther Methods Clin Dev,* 2022. **24**: p. 355-366.

[78] Wu, X., et al., A potent bispecific nanobody protects hACE2 mice against SARS-CoV-2 infection via intranasal administration. *Cell Rep,* 2021. **37**(3): p. 109869.

[79] Ye, G., et al., The Development of a Novel Nanobody Therapeutic for SARS-CoV-2. *bioRxiv,* 2020.

[80] Sun, D., et al., Potent neutralizing nanobodies resist convergent circulating variants of SARS-CoV-2 by targeting diverse and conserved epitopes. *Nat Commun,* 2021. **12**(1): p. 4676.

[81] Xiang, Y., et al., Versatile and multivalent nanobodies efficiently neutralize SARS-CoV-2. Science, 2020. **370**(6523): p. 1479-1484.

[82] Walter, J.D., et al., Biparatopic sybodies neutralize SARS-CoV-2 variants of concern and mitigate drug resistance. *EMBO Rep,* 2022. **23**(4): p. e54199.

[83] Dong, J., et al., Development of humanized tri-specific nanobodies with potent neutralization for SARS-CoV-2. *Sci Rep,* 2020. **10**(1): p. 17806.

[84] Wu, Y., et al., Identification of Human Single-Domain Antibodies against SARS-CoV-2. *Cell Host Microbe,* 2020. **27**(6): p. 891-898 e5.

[85] Wellner, A., et al., Rapid generation of potent antibodies by autonomous hypermutation in yeast. *Nat Chem Biol,* 2021. **17**(10): p. 1057-1064.

[86] Pymm, P., et al., Nanobody cocktails potently neutralize SARS-CoV-2 D614G N501Y variant and protect mice. *Proc Natl Acad Sci U S A,* 2021. **118**(19).

[87] Li, T., et al., A synthetic nanobody targeting RBD protects hamsters from SARS-CoV-2 infection. *Nat Commun,* 2021. **12**(1): p. 4635.

[88] Zhang, W., et al., An intracellular nanobody targeting T4SS effector inhibits Ehrlichia infection. *Proc Natl Acad Sci U S A,* 2021. **118**(18).

[89] Hanke, L., et al., A bispecific monomeric nanobody induces spike trimer dimers and neutralizes SARS-CoV-2 in vivo. *Nat Commun,* 2022. **13**(1): p. 155.

[90] Wang, Y., et al., A broad-spectrum nanobody targeting the C-terminus of the hepatitis B surface antigen for chronic hepatitis B infection therapy. *Antiviral Res,* 2022. **199**: p. 105265.

[91] Liu, X., et al., Preparation of a Nanobody Specific to Dectin 1 and Its Anti-inflammatory Effects on Fungal Keratitis. *Int J Nanomedicine,* 2022. **17**: p. 537-551.

[92] De Groof, T.W.M., et al., Targeting the latent human cytomegalovirus reservoir for T-cell-mediated killing with virus-specific nanobodies. *Nat Commun,* 2021. **12**(1): p. 4436.

[93] De Groof, T.W.M., et al., Nanobody-Targeted Photodynamic Therapy Selectively Kills Viral GPCR-Expressing Glioblastoma Cells. *Mol Pharm,* 2019. **16**(7): p. 3145-3156.

[94] Bernedo-Navarro, R.A., et al., Structural Basis for the Specific Neutralization of Stx2a with a Camelid Single Domain Antibody Fragment. *Toxins (Basel),* 2018. **10**(3).

[95] Ruano-Gallego, D., et al., Screening and purification of nanobodies from E. coli culture supernatants using the hemolysin secretion system. *Microb Cell Fact,* 2019. **18**(1): p. 47.

[96] Llauger, G., et al., Development of Nanobodies against Mal de Río Cuarto virus major viroplasm protein P9-1 for diagnostic sandwich ELISA and immunodetection. *Scientific Reports,* 2021. **11**(1): p. 20013.

[97] Gaiotto, T., et al., Nanobodies mapped to cross-reactive and divergent epitopes on A(H7N9) influenza hemagglutinin using yeast display. *Sci Rep,* 2021. **11**(1): p. 3126.

[98] Huo, J., et al., A potent SARS-CoV-2 neutralising nanobody shows therapeutic efficacy in the Syrian golden hamster model of COVID-19. *Nat Commun,* 2021. **12**(1): p. 5469.

[99] Esmagambetov, I.B., et al., Nanobodies Are Potential Therapeutic Agents for the Ebola Virus Infection. *Acta Naturae,* 2021. **13**(4): p. 53-63.

[100] Duan, H., et al., A novel intracellularly expressed NS5B-specific nanobody suppresses bovine viral diarrhea virus replication. *Vet Microbiol,* 2020. **240**: p. 108449.

[101] Cunha-Santos, C., et al., Inhibition of HIV replication through siRNA carried by CXCR4-targeted chimeric nanobody. *Cell Mol Life Sci,* 2020. **77**(14): p. 2859-2870.

[102] Jähnichen, S., et al., CXCR4 nanobodies (VHH-based single variable domains) potently inhibit chemotaxis and HIV-1 replication and mobilize stem cells. *Proc Natl Acad Sci U S A,* 2010. **107**(47): p. 20565-70.

[103] He, L., et al., Enhanced Ability of Oligomeric Nanobodies Targeting MERS Coronavirus Receptor-Binding Domain. *Viruses,* 2019. **11**(2).

[104] Zhao, G., et al., A Novel Nanobody Targeting Middle East Respiratory Syndrome Coronavirus (MERS-CoV) Receptor-Binding Domain Has Potent Cross-Neutralizing Activity and Protective Efficacy against MERS-CoV. *J Virol,* 2018. **92**(18).

[105] Wu, X., et al., A single-domain antibody inhibits SFTSV and mitigates virus-induced pathogenesis in vivo. *JCI Insight,* 2020. **5**(13).

[106] Koromyslova, A.D. and G.S. Hausman, Nanobodies Targeting Norovirus Capsid Reveal Functional Epitopes and Potential Mechanisms of Neutralization. *Biophysical Journal,* 2018. **114**(3): p. 219a-219a.

[107] Ruoff, K., et al., Structural Basis of Nanobodies Targeting the Prototype Norovirus. *Journal of Virology,* 2019. **93**(6).

[108] Ditlev, S.B., et al., Utilizing Nanobody Technology to Target Non-Immunodominant Domains of VAR2CSA. *Plos One,* 2014. **9**(1).

[109] Hufton, S.E., et al., The Breadth of Cross Sub-Type Neutralisation Activity of a Single Domain Antibody to Influenza Hemagglutinin Can Be Increased by Antibody Valency. *Plos One*, 2014. **9**(8).

[110] Gaiotto, T. and S.E. Hufton, Cross-Neutralising Nanobodies Bind to a Conserved Pocket in the Hemagglutinin Stem Region Identified Using Yeast Display and Deep Mutational Scanning. *Plos One,* 2016. **11**(10).

[111] Li, S.F., et al., Nanobody against the E7 oncoprotein of human papillomavirus 16. *Molecular Immunology,* 2019. **109**: p. 12-19.
[112] Zhang, W., et al., A novel intracellular nanobody against HPV16 E6 oncoprotein. *Clinical Immunology,* 2021. **225**.
[113] Vanmarsenille, C., et al., Nanobodies targeting conserved epitopes on the major outer membrane protein of Campylobacter as potential tools for control of Campylobacter colonization. *Veterinary Research,* 2017. **48**.
[114] Sparkes, A., et al., Novel half-life extended anti-MIF nanobodies protect against endotoxic shock. *Faseb Journal*, 2018. **32**(6): p. 3411-3422.
[115] Boons, E., et al., A stably expressed llama single-domain intrabody targeting Rev displays broad-spectrum anti-HIV activity. *Antiviral Research,* 2014. **112**: p. 91-102.

Index

G

H

I

L

M

N

O

P

R

S

T

U

V

W